Alcohol, Drugs and Health Promotion in Modern Ireland

SHANE BUTLER

IPA

INSTITUTE OF PUBLIC ADMINISTRATION

First published 2002
Institute of Public Administration
57-61 Lansdowne Road
Dublin 4
Ireland

ISBN 1 902448 77 4

British Library Cataloguing-in-Publication Data
A catalogue record for this book is available from the British Library

Cover design by Creative Inputs, Dublin
Typeset by Phototype-Set Ltd, Dublin
Printed by Future Print, Dublin

Contents

Preface

The completion of this book on Irish health policy relating to alcohol and illicit drugs reflects a long-standing professional interest on my part in this topic. Having trained originally as a sociologist and then as a psychiatric social worker, I wandered happily – albeit accidentally – into the addictions arena, first as a social worker and subsequently in my current academic post in Trinity College Dublin. While some may see the topic of alcohol and drug problems as highly specialist or peripheral to wider health policy concerns, this has never been my experience or perception. The main issues which arise in the analysis of alcohol and drug policy are, I believe, central to any analysis of healthcare systems, touching as they do upon the wisdom of expecting the healthcare system to treat away morbidity which is largely determined by individual lifestyle choices and by broader environmental factors. The practice of using psychoactive drugs for recreational purposes or as a means of coping with stress or tedium is ancient and almost universal, although knowledge of the negative consequences of such drug use is equally ancient and well-established. Health policy-making in this sphere is enormously complex, therefore, since it has to deal with abstract moral debate about drug use, popular opinion, economic and other interest group conflict, and of course with research developments in the biomedical and social sciences.

This book is my attempt to offer a detailed analysis of how our alcohol and drug policies have evolved from the mid-1940s up to 1996. I have resisted the temptation to bring the study right up to date: this is both because of difficulties in gathering detailed and accurate information on very recent events, and because I think readers may be better served by looking at the broad picture, rather than being distracted by what is topical in a policy area that easily lends itself to sensationalism. Those who work either in practice or in policy in the addictions field in Ireland will know that it is an area where strong views abound, where personality clashes are commonplace, and where ideological sparks fly. This being the case, it is almost inevitable that readers will take umbrage at certain of my arguments or conclusions; indeed there may be something in the book to annoy everybody. However, I can say, hand on heart, that I have tried my best to be accurate in gathering data and to be fair in my analysis and interpretation of the data. The fact that I have presented the alcohol and drug stories from a historical perspective, and within the theoretical context of health promotion, may help readers with current preoccupations with addiction matters to take a somewhat more detached view of the field. Whatever else, I hope readers are not bored!

I worked as a social worker at St Dymphna's Hospital (an addictions unit which was part of the larger St Brendan's Hospital, Grangegorman) between 1977 and 1983, and, in addition to giving me direct experience of work with clients with alcohol and drug problems, this whetted my appetite for studying the policy context of this aspect of the health service. R. D. Stevenson, who was Clinical Director of St Dymphna's, was a hard-working, practical clinician who became something of a legend amongst problem drinkers in Dublin. Sadly, he died quite soon after his retirement, but I am pleased to be able to record here my gratitude to him for what I learned while working with him during those years. All of my former colleagues in St Dymphna's contributed in various ways to my learning, and I recall particularly the energy and humour of Anna Lynch, Pearse Barnett, Judy Hickey and Bill Delaney.

The Department of Health and Children (although I have used the old title 'Department of Health' throughout the text) has financially supported the teaching of addiction studies at Trinity College Dublin for almost twenty years now. I am grateful for this financial support for the Diploma in Addiction Studies and the MSc in Drug and Alcohol Policy, just as I am grateful for the high degree of participation and challenge inherent in teaching mature students from a wide range of professional backgrounds on these courses. Anthony Coughlan supervised the doctoral thesis upon which this book is based, and other current and former colleagues at the Department of Social Studies in Trinity College – especially Vivienne Darling, Ruth Torode, Robbie Gilligan, Helen Buckley, Tony McCashin, Eoin O'Sullivan, Trish Walsh, Margaret Kirby, Gloria Kirwan and Alison Dye – have also been supportive of my research.

Des Corrigan of the School of Pharmacy at Trinity College, while always proclaiming himself to be to the right of Attila the Hun and completely out of sympathy with the liberal instincts of social scientists, has been extraordinarily generous in his support of addiction studies at Trinity, and it is a great pleasure to acknowledge his contribution to both my teaching and research. Since she came to the Department of Social Studies as a second addiction studies lecturer in 1997, Marguerite Woods has worked closely with me and I have gained considerably from her wisdom and experience. On the administrative front, Pam Isaacson has always been a model of calmness, of competence and of generosity; I am profoundly grateful to Pam for all her work on the addiction studies front and especially for her help with this book.

In thanking those who have helped by allowing me to do a research interview or to check specific points with them, I start by mentioning another former colleague, Noreen Kearney. Noreen was a member of both the Working Party on Drug Abuse and the Committee on Drug Education, as well as serving as a member of the Eastern Health Board when interesting policy events were taking place. She made available all her papers to me and patiently responded to my questions when I came back to her for information and clarification on innumerable occasions. Barry Cullen, who currently is Director of the Addiction Research Centre at Trinity College, was equally generous with his time in informing me about events in the south-inner city of Dublin during the years of the so-called 'opiate epidemic', as well as giving me access to his papers from this time.

I also wish to acknowledge the help of the following: Ruth Barrington, Joe Barry, Matt Bowden, Jim Comberton, Barry Desmond, Eugene Donoghue, Áine Flanagan, Paul Harrison, Paul Lavelle, Barbara Law, John McCormack, Denis Mullins, Fergus O'Kelly, Joe O'Rourke, Joe Power, Declan Roche, Tom Ryan, Martin Tansey, Dermot Walsh, Michael Walsh, and Mary Whelan. While I drew on the knowledge and experience of all of these informants, I must make it clear that they do not necessarily agree with any of the interpretations or conclusions contained in this study. When I was an undergraduate at UCD, I took a course in social policy which was taught with great gusto by Helen Burke; years later, I sought her guidance for the present study and she responded with typical generosity and enthusiasm, for which I am most grateful.

I would like to acknowledge the financial support towards the publication of this book which came from the Research Maintenance Grant Scheme of the Dean of Research at Trinity College Dublin, and the editorial and publishing assistance of Tony McNamara, Eleanor Ashe, Jim Power and Hannah Ryan at the Institute of Public Administration.

Finally, I thank my family for their forbearance with my preoccupation with this project. My wife, Phil, and my daughters, Emer and Gráinne, have been generally interested and supportive. My son, Kilian, offered quite specific but somewhat lurid advice as to the cover design – thanks anyway!

Shane Butler
August 2002

Alcohol, Drugs and Health Promotion: Introduction

The health and social problems associated with the consumption of alcohol and of illicit drugs have long been causes of concern in international public health circles. Empirical studies (Bruun et al, 1975; Davies and Walsh, 1983; Edwards et al, 1994) have revealed that from the middle of the twentieth century alcohol consumption has increased in most Western societies, as have many indicators of alcohol-associated morbidity and mortality. Both national and international health authorities have sought during this period to devise treatment responses for those already experiencing problems and prevention strategies to reduce the incidence of drinking problems. Similarly, there has been a major expansion in the range of illicit drugs widely available and widely used. This, to some extent, is a by-product of developments in the area of science and technology since drugs, like other commodities, may now be transported easily and quickly around the world away from their geographical source, and synthetic drugs may equally easily be manufactured in relatively unsophisticated laboratories. The growth in the international trade in drugs may also be explained sociologically as just one example of the wider phenomenon of *globalisation,* which refers to political and economic processes facilitating international trade and diminishing the importance of border controls. While health authorities have been concerned with the provision of treatment and rehabilitation services for those who become dependent on drugs or who have other drug-related health problems, a great deal of public attention has also focused on the drug control or supply-side policies which have been set in place internationally. These include the use of a variety of technical and legal measures which are intended to prevent drug trafficking, and in the United States of America where they have been pursued with particular zeal these activities have been popularly described as a War on Drugs.

The present study is concerned with Irish health care policy and practice in relation to alcohol and drug problems in the post-World War II period, from 1945 to 1996. One of the central issues to be explored is the tension between treatment and prevention in these two closely related areas of public health. The tension referred to involves decision-making as to the relative allocation of time, energy and, above all, resources to tackling these problems. In strictly logical terms, it seems invalid to devote the lion's share of scarce resources to curative services, while there are environmental or lifestyle factors which contribute to the incidence and prevalence of ill-health but which are largely ignored by health policy. In terms of practical reality, however, those critics who maintain that what we have in Ireland is an 'illness service' rather than a health service, can justify this allegation by simple reference to the manner in which resources are allocated within the Irish health care system. The *Commission on Health Funding* (1989) reported that health expenditure as a proportion of GNP doubled, from 4.8 to 9.6 per cent, between 1960 and 1988; and Wiley (1998) has shown that while the share of GNP/GDP devoted to non-capital health expenditure has declined between 1990 and 1996, this still – because of economic growth during this period – represented a funding increase in real terms. However, there has been no significant diversion of funding from curative to preventive services, and institutional services (mainly consisting of general hospitals, as well as the largely institution-based psychiatric and mental handicap services) continue to account for about 70 per cent of total non-capital expenditure. General hospitals alone have continued to account for about half of total non-capital expenditure.

In tracing and comparing the evolution of Irish alcohol and drug policies from a health perspective, therefore, a major aim of this book is to identify the extent to which policy makers have sought to combine and co-ordinate all elements of policy into a balanced and rational whole. In each case it is clear that prevention policies cannot be expected to function effectively if they are solely the function of health care institutions; instead, effective preventive policies depend upon multisectoral collaboration, in which other institutions (in the industrial, financial, legal, educational and other spheres) combine with health care interests to reduce the incidence of alcohol and drug-related problems. For instance, it is difficult to see how Irish health care institutions could expect to reduce or contain the incidence of drug-related problems, if the criminal justice system did not simultaneously enforce the legal measures which are aimed at curbing the supply of illicit substances.

Although the prevention of illness and the promotion of health might generally be perceived as being socially desirable objectives, it would be naïve to assume that public health is such a dominant value in society that multisectoral collaboration is guaranteed or that other institutions would automatically subordinate their own interests to the health interest. No such assumption of rationality or consensus will be made in this book. Instead, the intention is to explore empirically the extent to which policy making in this area has succeeded over the period studied in drawing together the various institutional strands which have a bearing on the prevention of dependence and other alcohol and drug related problems.

While it is obviously important to maintain a clear focus on the co-ordination of public policy at the level of central government, there is a risk in doing so of presenting a picture which exaggerates the extent to which the policy-making process is a *top-down* activity. Academic work on this topic over the past twenty years has clearly indicated the dubious validity of models which suggest that policy is invariably made at a high or governmental level and then passed down for execution or implementation to lower bodies. Evolving ideas, such as those which look at policy making and policy implementation through organisational networks, have argued that the policy-making process is more complex than this, and that the distinction between policy formulation and policy execution is not as clear-cut as it was previously considered to be. On the contrary, it is argued that those who implement policy, and who may be at a relatively low level in their organisational hierarchy, are frequently involved in the type of bargaining, negotiation and general interaction which in itself is characteristic of policy making. Applying these ideas to the alcohol and drugs arena in Ireland, one is reminded that health policy makers are not solely to be found in the Department of Health or other central government departments, but that health board workers, professional bodies, voluntary organisations and other community groupings may all be considered from this perspective.

The health promotion paradigm which will be used as the underlying conceptual framework for this study combines both the top-down and the bottom-up policy approaches: the former emphasises the importance of co-ordinating intersectoral policy activity at central government level, while the latter, both descriptively and prescriptively, argues for more participatory and communitarian inputs to the policy process. This health promotion paradigm will now be considered in detail.

Health promotion

From the moment of its establishment in 1946 the World Health Organisation (WHO) was determined that its focus should not be exclusively on the provision of curative services for those already ill. In its foundation charter the WHO declared that:

> Health is a state of complete physical, mental and social well-being and not merely the absence of disease and infirmity.[1]

This definition, so utopian as to prompt one early critic to compare it with a state of perfection, 'such as was enjoyed perhaps by archangels and by Adam before the Fall',[2] presaged the broad approach to health which has been a feature of WHO activities ever since. In an era which was characterised by technological advances in the specialised areas of clinical medicine and surgery, the WHO has consistently championed the development of primary health services which are flexible and readily accessible to local communities, and has reiterated the importance for public health of basic environmental factors, such as housing, sanitation and nutrition.

The concept of health promotion has evolved gradually from the early ideals of the WHO and has been consistently aimed at enabling people to achieve health as it was originally defined in the foundation charter. The phrase 'health promotion' appears to have been first used in a Canadian policy document, *A New Perspective on the Health of Canadians,* which was published by Marc Lalonde, the Canadian Minister of National Health and Welfare, in 1974.[3] The WHO does not operate as a free-standing or isolated international health organisation, but functions as a forum where ideas from researchers and policy makers from all over the world are debated, codified and thereby given a new authority and status. Emerging ideas on health promotion were given such an authoritative status in the WHO's *Strategy for Health for All by the Year 2000* which was drawn up at an international conference on primary health care at Alma Ata in 1977.[4] However, for the purpose of this study, the clearest statement of what the aims of health promotion are and of the means most likely to achieve these aims is that contained in the *Ottawa Charter for Health Promotion* of 1986.[5]

The Ottawa Charter, which was drawn up jointly by the WHO and the Canadian Public Health Association, starts by defining health in precisely the same positive terms as those cited above from the WHO foundation charter. It anticipates criticism that health ought not to be seen as an end in itself by suggesting that health should be 'seen as a resource for life, not the objective of living'. Most importantly, the Ottawa Charter identifies five overlapping and interlinked tasks which policy makers must undertake if health promotion is to become a reality. In summary, policy makers must undertake the following:

• **Build healthy public policy** – sometimes referred to colloquially as 'health-proofing' public policy, this consists of putting health on the agenda of policy makers in all sectors of government so as to ensure safer and healthier goods and services, healthier public services and cleaner and more enjoyable environments.

- *Create supportive environments* – this entails a recognition of the inter-dependence of people and their environments, on the basis that if human beings do not maintain healthy living and working environments, these environments will not in turn sustain and maximise human health.
- *Strengthen community action* – health promotion is based on the idea that lay people should be facilitated to increase control over their own health; thus, rather than depending solely on central government initiatives or the formal activity of health care bodies and professionals, local communities should participate fully in identifying and developing strategies for the promotion of health in their own areas.
- *Develop personal skills* – this reflects the view that individuals may to a large extent determine their own health patterns by virtue of their 'lifestyles' or the choices they make in terms of diet, exercise, drug use and other such behaviours; by being informed and by enhancing their decision-making skills, people may optimise their health.
- *Reorient health services* – while the rhetoric of health promotion has a very positive focus on the prevention of illness and on maximising the quality of life, the reality is that the traditional activities of health services, and the professionals who work within them, have been concentrated on the care and treatment of those already ill; if health promotion is to become a reality, health service professionals must be re-educated to take on the broad, holistic views and activities implicit in this new approach.

From an analytical perspective, health promotion may be regarded as seeking to incorporate two principal, and potentially conflicting, components: the first of these is the *individualistic* component which refers to individual behavioural choices or lifestyles and their impact on health, while the second is the *structural* component which refers to the impact of socio-economic and other environmental factors on the health of wider populations. Later in this chapter some of the main criticisms of health promotion will be discussed; suffice it to say at this point that if health promotion consisted solely of an individualistic approach, as did traditional health education, it would evoke even sharper criticism on the grounds that it ignored the limitations on individual choice, particularly amongst economically and politically disadvantaged groups, and thereby constituted a form of 'victim blaming'.

For some authors on health promotion, these aspirations and strategies constitute a 'new public health'.[6] The use of this phrase involves a conscious harking back to the radical improvements in public health which were achieved in urbanised and industrialised areas during the nineteenth century, through the introduction of a range of environmental measures. However, where the old public health involved the adaptation of the physical environment – such as the provision of clean drinking water and sanitation, improved housing standards, and food hygiene – health promotion, or the new public health, has a much broader and more ambitious vision of the environment which incorporates cultural, economic and political factors. Clearly, therefore, the task of realising health promotion ideals is complex and formidable.

This summary account of health promotion is not intended as an uncritical espousal of the paradigm, nor is it intended to suggest that Irish drug and alcohol policy over the past fifty years *ought* to have conformed to this paradigm. The latter suggestion would be absurd since the health promotion concept, while not entirely new, has only evolved in its present form since the mid-1970s. However, it will be used here as the conceptual framework for examining the curative/preventive tension in drug and alcohol policies and services in post-war Ireland, since it contains within a single coherent policy outline reference to all of the relevant major factors and issues. It is hoped that the health promotion paradigm will prove to be a useful vehicle for the presentation and analysis of drug and alcohol data, and, in turn, that the findings of this study will provide a basis for testing the general validity and practicability of health promotion ideas.

Health promotion in Ireland

While health promotion has continued to be elaborated and refined at international level, particularly within the World Health Organisation, this paradigm has also gained considerable currency in Ireland. The *Health for All by the Year 2000* document was further developed by WHO Europe, as a result of which 38 specific targets for its successful implementation were identified. In Ireland acceptance of these health promotion ideals was explicitly expressed for the first time in a 1986 policy document from the Department of Health entitled *Health: The Wider Dimensions*. This policy document was heavily influenced by the ideas contained in *Health for All by the Year 2000*, although in a postscript the novelty and radicalism of the proposals were acknowledged in the statement that: 'The cynical and fatalistic will possibly dismiss such an approach as a grand design incapable of being achieved'.[7] In 1987 a health promotion group which had been working under the auspices of the Health Education Bureau

(HEB) published its report, *Promoting Health Through Public Policy,* which again summarised many of the evolving health promotion ideas. Essentially, this report reiterated the view that public health was unlikely to be improved significantly by further technological advances in curative medicine, and it decried what it saw as an exclusively curative ethos within Irish health services, arguing that:

> The present role of the Minister for Health is primarily one of providing services to deal with sickness rather than promoting health ... We recommend new statutory provisions expanding the role of the Minister for Health to being responsible for the promotion of the health of the Irish people in addition to providing traditional health services.[8]

The report also recommended that this redefined role of the Minister for Health should be reflected in structural changes in the Department of Health, that the Minister should be statutorily required to produce regular health promotion plans and, finally, that a statutory Health Promotion Council should be established.

While no statutory changes resulted from these recommendations, they did bear considerable fruit. Ironically, since *Promoting Health Through Public Policy* emanated from the HEB, this agency was abolished in 1988 and replaced by a new section within the Department of Health, the Health Promotion Unit. An Advisory Council on Health Promotion was also established, as was a cabinet sub-committee on health promotion, chaired by the Minister for Health and consisting of the Ministers for Education, Energy, Labour, Agriculture and the Environment. The final development in what was seen as a new, national health promotion structure was the funding by the Department of Health of a Chair in Health Promotion in the medical school of University College, Galway.

Such was the centrality and apparent public acceptability of health promotion during the 1990s that in 1994, when the Department of Health launched its four-year strategy *Shaping a Healthier Future,* no public or political controversy was aroused by the explicit and implicit use of health promotion concepts in this highly-publicised document. The WHO influence is clearly discernible, for example, in the contention that:

> A central aspect of the Strategy is to reorient the health services towards a health promotion approach based on encouraging people to take responsibility for their own health and on providing the environmental support necessary to achieve this. Many of the targets in this Strategy depend crucially on a co-ordinated and integrated approach to health promotion.[9]

Finally, in 1995 the Department of Health published a specific policy document, *A Health Promotion Strategy: making the healthier choice the easier choice,*[10] which largely reiterated the ideas of *Shaping a Healthier Future* and which identified goals and targets to be aimed for in the realisation of its health promotional ideals. This 1995 policy document contained a brief section on alcohol and substance misuse in the broader context of 'risk factors and lifestyle', which will be referred to later in this book.

Health policy-making structures and processes

While health promotion appears *prima facie* to be an excellent notion, it is not difficult to see beyond its idealism to the practical and philosophical difficulties inherent in this paradigm. Cultural or ideological objections to what is sometimes seen as the overweening influence of medicine in everyday life, or state paternalism in relation to healthy lifestyles, will be discussed in the next section of this chapter, but this section will look at the practical difficulties which arise in the creation of policy-making structures and processes capable of translating the rhetoric of the Ottawa Charter into real policy achievements.

Firstly, in relation to healthy public policy, one must ask whether it could ever be possible to achieve the degree of intersectoral co-ordination at central government level that would be necessary for the building of such policy. In order to gain a preliminary understanding of the range and roles of Irish central government departments which have a function in relation to alcohol and drugs, and in order to appreciate the complexity and difficulty involved in co-ordinating such a disparate range of activities, Table 1 sets out the major departmental functions relevant to this particular area of health promotion.

In the case of illicit drugs, there are fewer departments involved in the policy-making process and there is less cultural ambivalence about this type of drug use, which may assist in the co-ordination of comprehensive drug policies; however, the task of policy making in this sphere is still far from simple. In the case of alcohol, there is considerable and obvious potential for a conflict of interests between departments whose approaches to this topic may vary radically; the Department of Health might be committed, for example, to improving public health through a reduction of alcohol consumption levels in Irish society, while other departments (Finance, Enterprise and Employment, the Revenue Commissioners, Agriculture, Food and Forestry, for example) might be primarily concerned with strengthening the drinks industry so as to maximise revenue for the exchequer or create additional jobs.

Baggot, in his study of British alcohol policy, has described the process

Table 1: Role of central Government Departments* in relation to alcohol and drugs

Department of Health	plays a co-ordinating role for all other departments in the prevention of alcohol and drug problems, as well as being directly responsible for treatment and rehabilitation policy.
Department of Education	has overall policy responsibility for health education for school-going children.
Department of Justice	has policy responsibility for liquor licensing laws, and for law enforcement in this area and in relation to drink-driving legislation and misuse of drugs legislation.
Revenue Commissioners	collect excise duties on alcoholic beverages and, through the customs service, combat smuggling of alcohol and illicit drugs.
Department of Finance	as part of its overall finance function, sets alcohol taxes and is concerned with revenue and job-creation aspects of drinks and pharmaceutical industry, and with costs of health services.
Department of Enterprise and Employment	seek to develop the drinks industry, both in its manufacturing and retailing aspects, and to promote the pharmaceutical industry.
Department of Tourism and Trade	has an interest in the retailing of beverages in the context of its wider concern for the provision of services for tourists, and in the export of alcohol and pharmaceutical products
Department of the Environment	has policy responsibility for drink-driving legislation.

* Irish central government departments as they were in 1996

where an individual department pursues its own policy agenda in a manner which is either indifferent or inimical to the agenda of other departments as 'departmentalism', and has underlined the difficulties inherent in moving from traditional governmental activity of this type towards health promotion ideals.[11] In their study of the co-ordination of alcohol and tobacco policies in the United Kingdom, Harrison and Tether have also identified departmentalism as a major obstacle to the type of policy co-ordination which would appear to be called for under the rubric of healthy public policy.[12] They examine three specific models of policy co-ordination which they consider most relevant to this task. The first, a rational-comprehensive or *corporate* model, whereby all central government policy activity would be brought into line with an agreed, dominant policy objective such as health promotion, is dismissed on the grounds that it is unrealistic and impracticable. Harrison and Tether conclude that, in real governmental affairs, consensus of this type between departments simply does not exist. The second model, known as *partisan mutual adjustment,* acknowledges that government departments and other agencies and interest groups are partisan, that is they tend to have distinctive and sometimes conflicting policy agendas; in practice, however, these bodies interact and bargain informally and incrementally, and in so doing create policy which is mutually acceptable, although falling short of what purists or advocates of the corporate approach might see as the optimum.

Harrison and Tether are critical of partisan mutual adjustment on the grounds that it is excessively conservative and *laissez faire,* and is highly unlikely to result in policy co-ordination which would be deemed satisfactory from a health perspective. Therefore, they argue prescriptively for a third model, the *organisational networks* approach, which is something of a compromise between the two extremes represented by the other two models. The organisational networks model of policy co-ordination is more systematic, coherent and rational than partisan mutual adjustment, although still falling considerably short of the ideals of the corporate or rational comprehensive model. Essentially, it is suggested that across the array of organisational stakeholders involved in an area of common policy interest there are identifiable groupings or networks which communicate and negotiate on an on-going basis. Typically, these networks consist of specialist sub-units or personnel rather than total organisations: in the context of this study such sub-units might include the Health Promotion Unit of the Department of Health, the Drug Squad of the Garda Síochána, or the Youth Affairs or Psychological Service sections of the Department of Education. While the structure of the network is relatively fragile and tenuous, it has the capacity, if those involved are sufficiently committed and skilled, to create and sustain a reasonable amount of policy co-ordination.

Of the three policy co-ordination models presented by Harrison and Tether, it would appear that organisational networks is the model which is the most realistic and practical for the achievement of health promotion. Much of the literature which advocates health promotion, and this would include the Irish policy documents referred to above, has done so in a superficial, almost evangelical way, which tacitly assumes that public policy making is a rational process and that this rationality will suffice to achieve the successful delivery of health promotion. The most obvious example of this rational/managerial bias is to be found in the tendency of policy documents to set great store on the identification of quantified goals and targets which are to be achieved by a specified date; such target-setting usually fails to acknowledge the fact that there is no evidence of overall, intersectoral consensus on the desirability of health promotion, and frequently has no accompanying strategy which appears likely to achieve these goals and targets.

An interesting and highly relevant development in public administration in Ireland which took place almost at the end of the study period was the establishment by Government of the *Strategic Management Initiative* (SMI) in 1994. This initiative, which was heavily influenced by public management developments in New Zealand and Australia, was largely based on the view that the achievement of important public policy objectives frequently demanded a level of intersectoral collaboration which did not routinely exist in Ireland's fragmented and 'departmentalist' central governmental system. An important aim of SMI, therefore, was the establishment of structures and processes to manage these 'cross-cutting' issues, with explicit reference being made for the first time in this country to an organisational networks style of policy formulation and implementation.[13] This development, to some extent, influenced the decision to set up both a National Drug Strategy Team at central government level and Local Drugs Task Forces at community level, developments which will be discussed towards the end of this book.

A second potential complication of the policy process which must be considered here concerns the 'bottom-up' style of policy making inherent in the Ottawa Charter's identification of community action as a necessary ingredient of health promotion. The concept of community is, of course, notoriously vague and ill-defined, yet it is one which in the social policy area is constantly deferred to and of which much is expected. In the context of health promotion, however, it appears quite clear that community action refers to participation of local people in activities which maximise health, prevent the incidence of health problems and abate existing problems. Ideas of this kind may also be found in the McKinsey Report upon which the administrative structures of Ireland's regional health boards were established following the Health Act, 1970.[14] The Community Care Programme, one of three programmes within the conventional structure of the health boards, was not merely intended to provide for the delivery of health and social services in non-institutional settings, but was also intended to foster and encourage local participation in such services. There is also a strong tradition of voluntarism in social services in Ireland, part of which at least was rooted in the principle of *subsidiarity*; this is a tenet of Roman Catholic social teaching which argues that, as far as possible, the performance of important societal functions should be carried out by bodies lesser than the State – such as the family, local community groups, vocational groups or others. The period from 1987 to 1996, the last nine years of the half-century studied in this thesis, has been characterised by an emphasis on *social partnership* in the management of the economy; much of the credit for the unprecedented economic growth during this period is given to this conscious and explicit utilisation of a partnership model of public governance in which sectional interests and local groupings work together to achieve common social and economic gains.

Paradoxically, however, there has long been a perception that modern Ireland is characterised by a high degree of administrative centralisation, and it would be naïve to overlook the generally sceptical views of analysts and commentators on the level of communitarian or grass-roots participation in Irish public life for much of the period studied here. Lee, for example, has argued that despite the image of Ireland as a country characterised by strong, self-reliant rural communities (an image usually associated with the vision of Eamon de Valera), the period since self-government in 1921 has in fact been marked by continuous centralisation of a political, administrative and geographic nature.[15] Similarly, Barrington, a persistent critic of what he saw as a breakdown of local democracy in Ireland, wrote in 1982:

> There is increasing acceptance in European countries that three great diseases of the modern state are alienation of the people, amoral centralised corporatism, and congested government. I think there can be no doubt but that, in this country, those three diseases are far advanced.[16]

Perhaps the most plausible explanation for this centralisation of government in modern Ireland is offered by Garvin, who suggests that during the transition to self-government in 1922 both sides in the Civil War were distrustful of the elaborate system of local government which had been inherited from the British. He argues specifically that: 'Neither side truly believed in secular participant local democracy and both foresaw that such participation would, if unfettered, lead to a widespread corruption of public life.'[17] Obviously, therefore, the present study of alcohol and drug policy making must not presume that Irish health authorities are enthusiasts for community participation in health policy matters, whatever the current view of the World Health Organisation on this subject.

It is important before leaving this issue to refer to the tradition of self-help which is particularly strong in the alcohol and drugs field; the original work of Alcoholics Anonymous (AA), established in the USA in 1935, has influenced the creation of a plethora of similar 'fellowships' in the addictions area. AA and the other related fellowships may, on the face of it, be considered as constituting a form of community action; they are enduring mutual associations of persons with a common experience, they are non-professional by their nature, do not seek or accept outside funding and their sole concern is to provide help and support for those affected by these problems. AA and its related fellowships have been solely concerned with curative-type activities (although they might not be comfortable with such a description) but it is important in the present study to explore what the consequences of this curative activity have been for the wider area of prevention and health promotion, and perhaps for Irish culture generally.

A third institutional or structural impediment to health promotion which will be alluded to here concerns the role of the medical profession and, to a lesser extent, other health care professionals and institutions. What must be borne in mind is that health promotion policies did not originate within these traditional groupings or institutions and that, while not couched in the sharply critical language of some well-known critiques of medicine, they are nonetheless fundamentally critical of curative medicine. The existing health care system is dominated by doctors who have been trained, intensively and expensively, in traditional curative medicine and who on a daily basis are busily engaged in the treatment of patients with real, and often life-threatening, illnesses; such doctors may not routinely be aware of health promotion at all. While some clinicians may contribute actively to health promotion campaigns in their specific area of interest and expertise (respiratory physicians are frequently involved in campaigns against tobacco, for instance), by and large they are too caught up with the treatment of patients to devote much time to this, and they would certainly not agree to a radical reorientation of health services if this involved a transfer of resources from their hospitals and clinics in favour of preventive activities. The Ottawa Charter's recommendation that health services should be reoriented is clearly sensible if one is in favour of health promotion; what is not so clear is whether or how the existing health services can be reoriented in the absence of strong support from this powerful and respected group of traditionally trained clinicians.

Ideological and cultural objections to health promotion

Apart from these structural or institutional impediments to health promotion, there are at the level of abstract ideas some common objections or criticisms which will be looked at here. The most fundamental critique of health promotion discourse and practice is that which comes from academic sociologists and which argues that health promotion is essentially a moral or cultural enterprise masquerading as objective science. An early example of such sociological work was Zola's seminal paper on 'Medicine as an institution of social control' (Zola, 1972) which argued – to some extent before health promotion had got into its current stride – that ever-increasing areas of life were being drawn into the ambit of medicine without clear and open debate as to the value systems inherent in this process. Zola summarised his fears about this expansion of medicine to cover all aspects of life by citing a colleague, Freidson, who had suggested that: 'A profession and a society which are so concerned with physical and functional wellbeing as to sacrifice civil liberty and moral integrity must inevitably press for a "scientific" environment similar to that provided laying hens on progressive chicken farms – hens who produce eggs industriously and have no disease or other cares'.[18] As health promotion has been developed in the manner described above, sociological critique has also expanded to look critically at the assumption that health is axiomatically a dominant value and that environment must be restructured and individual lifestyles altered in the interests of health.

Some of the more polemical objections to health promotion are expressed in libertarian terms, with this new approach to public health being described as a form of state paternalism or 'nannyism' which intrudes to an unacceptable extent into the lives of individuals and overrides what would be seen as the more important social value of maximising individual personal choices. Skrabanek, an Irish community health academic who was consistently opposed to health promotion and tended to refer to it provocatively as 'health fascism', wrote in the mid-1980s:

> Even if the enforcement of a uniform 'healthy' lifestyle were possible, would not the evil of allowing others to decide what is good for us be a sufficient reason for subverting such [a] society?[19]

Ideological objections of this kind, published in British or international journals, may perhaps be considered to be of minimal influence on policy developments in Ireland; yet it is important to point out that such objections – while expressed in secular philosophical terms – have strong theological resonances with recent Irish history. The influence of the Roman Catholic Church on social policy in Ireland has long been acknowledged and researched, and Whyte's classic study of church-state relations contains a detailed account of the infamous 'mother and child scheme' episode of 1951.[20] Opposition to this health scheme came from two main sources, the Irish medical profession and the Roman Catholic Hierarchy; the latter expressed its opposition to the proposed health scheme in terms of the social teaching of the church, which disapproved of state health services (and indeed the state generally) playing an overweening role in the lives of citizens. The role and influence of the Roman Catholic Church in the sphere of alcohol and drug policies must therefore be examined continuously throughout this study, and, in particular, it must be remembered that some aspects of health promotion policy may be ideologically or 'doctrinally' repugnant to this powerful institution.

Before leaving the topic of potential church opposition to health promotion, it is of interest to note that about the time of Skrabanek's criticism cited above, the then Roman Catholic Bishop of Limerick, Dr Newman, explicitly criticised health promotion policy in Ireland, linking it to the earlier mother and child scheme controversy, and viewing it as a new totalitarian development which had to be resisted. Dr Newman referred to the HEB publication, *Promoting Health Through Public Policy,* and concluded:

> Some day one could expect – if government were to be sole arbiter – an injunction that one should eat porridge but not cornflakes for one's breakfast ... Already the 'thin end of the wedge' as regards that kind of thing has come with the announcement by the Minister for Health that a Bill to control smoking in public places is shortly to be introduced; also that work is proceeding on controls over the promotion and advertising of such products as tobacco, alcohol and unsuitable food (cf. *Irish Times,* 29 May, 1987). It is genuinely hard to know where it will all end.[21]

In addition to ideological objections of the foregoing variety which fundamentally challenge the ethics of health promotion, there are a number of other criticisms of this policy approach which question the accuracy and the effectiveness of much of the healthy lifestyles information. In summary, such criticisms argue that the advice given to the public on topics such as food and alcohol consumption, drug use, sexual behaviour and other potentially health-related activity is of doubtful scientific validity; it is suggested that advice of this kind exaggerates the risks involved, conceals the fact that most of those persuaded to change their behaviour will derive little, if any, benefit from such change and, finally, that the entire business of lifestyle direction is better understood as a social movement than as a scientific enterprise.

Nadelmann, a contemporary critic of American drug policy, has argued, for instance, that the risks associated with illicit drug use have been greatly exaggerated in that society's drug education programmes, and that:

> The government, in its efforts to discourage people from using illicit drugs, has encouraged and perpetuated these misconceptions not just in its rhetoric but also in its purportedly educational materials. Only by reading between the lines can the facts be discerned that the vast majority of Americans who have used illicit drugs have done so in moderation, that relatively few have suffered negative short-term consequences, and given available evidence, that few are likely to suffer long-term harm.[22]

Of particular relevance to the present study, which looks at both alcohol and drug policy, is the provocative contention of Szasz, the well-known anti-psychiatrist and libertarian, that attempts to distinguish between acceptable drugs, such as alcohol, and unacceptable drugs, such as heroin, in terms of the science of chemistry are no more sensible than seeking to use chemistry to distinguish between ordinary tap water and 'holy' water.[23] The distinction in both cases, he maintains, is one of cultural ritual or ceremonial.

Finally, in this context, it should be noted that recent advice to the public concerning what are 'safe' levels of alcohol consumption is also not without its critics. Academic commentators, such as Skrabanek, have argued that the public is misled as to the scientific validity of the methods whereby 'experts' arrive at these recommendations, while researchers employed by the drinks industry have described this entire business as 'neo-prohibitionism' or 'pseudo-science'.

Aims of this book

Against the background described above, this book sets out to answer the following questions:

- What were the main health and social policies pursued in relation to alcohol and illicit drugs in Ireland in the post-war period?
- Which were the main interest groups or stakeholders within the policy-making process; how did they interact and to what extent was this process co-ordinated by either national or regional health authorities?
- What lessons concerning the general practicability of health promotion may be learned from this study of alcohol and drugs?

Structure of this book

The lay-out of this book consists of two main sections, one dealing with alcohol policy and the other dealing with illicit drug policy, while the final chapter combines analytically the conclusions from these two sections.

The importance of the final chapter (Chapter Eight) lies in the fact that it is here that the basic question concerning the feasibility of the health promotion paradigm in Ireland will be most sharply considered, and it is here also that recommendations will be made for a reframing of health promotion in a style which reflects the Irish situation.

NOTES

1. Cited in A. Clare, *Psychiatry in Dissent: Controversial Issues in Thought and Practice.* (London: Tavistock, 1976), p.9.

2. A. Lewis, 'Health as a Social Concept', *British Journal of Sociology, 4* (1953), p.110.

3. M. Lalonde, *A New Perspective on the Health of Canadians.* (Ottawa: Information Canada, 1974).

4. World Health Organisation, *Primary Health Care (Report of the International Conference on Primary Health Care, Alma Ata, 6-12 September, 1978).* (Geneva: WHO, 1978).

5. World Health Organisation, *Ottawa Charter for Health Promotion.* (Geneva: WHO, 1986).

6. For the use of this phrase by proponents of health promotion, see J. Ashton and H. Seymour, *The New Public Health: The Liverpool Experience.* (Milton Keynes: Open University Press, 1988); for a more critical sociological use of the phrase, see A. Petersen and D. Lupton, *The New Public Health: Health and Self in the Age of Risk.* (London: Sage, 1996).

7. *Health: The Wider Dimensions (A Consultative Statement on Health Policy).* (Dublin: Department of Health, 1986), Appendix 1.

8. *Promoting Health Through Public Policy.* (Dublin: Health Education Bureau, 1987), p.56.

9. *Shaping a Healthier Future: A Strategy for Effective Health-Care in the 1990s.* (Dublin: Stationery Office, 1994), p.48.

10. *A Health Promotion Strategy: making the healthier choice the easier choice.* (Dublin: Department of Health, 1995).

11. R. Baggot, *Alcohol, Politics and Social Policy.* (Aldershot: Gower, 1990).

12. L. Harrison and P. Tether, 'The Co-Ordination of UK Policy on Alcohol and Tobacco: The significance of organisational networks', *Policy and Politics, 15* (1987), pp 77-90.

13. D. Byrne et al, *Strategic Management in the Irish Civil Service: a review drawing on the experience in New Zealand and Australia.* (Special issue of *Administration,* vol. 43, no.2, 1995); *Delivering Better Government: a programme of change for the Irish Civil Service.* (Dublin: Stationery Office, 1996); R. Boyle, *The Management of Cross-Cutting Issues.* (Dublin: Institute of Public Administration, 1999).

14. McKinsey and Co., *Towards Better Health Care.* (Dublin: Department of Health, 1970/71).

15. J. Lee, 'Centralisation and Community', in J. Lee (ed.), *Ireland: Towards a Sense of Place.* (Cork University Press, 1985), pp 84-101.

16.   T. Barrington, 'Whatever Happened to Irish Government?', *Administration, 30* (1982), p.107.

17.   T. Garvin, *1922: The Birth of Irish Democracy.* (Dublin: Gill and Macmillan, 1996), p.90.

18.   I. Zola, 'Medicine as an Institution of Social Control', *Sociological Review, 20* (1973), p.503.

19.   P. Skrabanek, 'Preventive Medicine and Morality', *The Lancet (i)* (1986), p.144.

20.   J. Whyte, *Church and State in Modern Ireland, 1923-1979 (2nd ed.).* (Dublin: Gill and Macmillan, 1980).

21.   J. Newman, *Puppets of Utopia: Can Irish democracy be taken for granted?* (Dublin: Four Courts Press, 1987), p.75.

22.   E. Nadelmann, 'U.S. Drug Policy: A Bad Export', *Foreign Policy, 70* (1988), p.93.

23.   T. Szasz, *Ceremonial Chemistry: The Ritual Persecution of Drugs, Addicts and Pushers.* (London: Routledge and Kegan Paul, 1975).

Alcoholism: The Disease Concept in the Ascendant 1945-1972

Irish alcohol policy: the historical and sociological context

The presentation of a detailed account of Irish alcohol policy in the post-World War II era will be more intelligible if set in a historical and socio-cultural context; hence this brief introduction which will attempt to identify the most salient policy issues emerging from a review of alcohol policy in Ireland since the mid-nineteenth century.

During the mid-nineteenth century, the 'social scientists' of this period, notably the members of the *Statistical and Social Inquiry Society of Ireland* (SSISI),[1] were preoccupied with alcohol-related problems about which they saw themselves as offering dispassionate and value-free policy advice. The political impact of such advice appears to have been negligible, however, and by far the greatest influence on public opinion and public policy at this time was that of the church-based temperance groups. Historical studies[2] are agreed that the well-known temperance campaign started by the Capuchin priest Fr Theobald Mathew during the 1840s was largely based upon the charismatic qualities of its founder and so did not survive his death; however, its successor, the Pioneer Total Abstinence Association which was founded in 1898, was firmly institutionalised within the Roman Catholic Church in Ireland and remained so throughout the twentieth century. Drawing upon the sociological work of Levine (1992),[3] it is clear that Ireland was never a 'temperance culture' in the sense of having a large and enduring temperance movement based upon the idea that alcohol was inherently evil and advocating prohibition as an acceptable policy measure. Levine, in fact, suggests that temperance cultures of this kind are uniquely associated with Protestantism. The Irish Pioneer movement, while acknowledging the potential and actual harm resulting from alcohol consumption, reflected the mainstream Roman Catholic view of alcohol as inherently good, being one of God's gifts – albeit a gift which could be abused and which some people might voluntarily refuse for religious motives.

19

It is also clear from historical research[4] into the public lunatic asylums which the British government in Ireland established from 1817 onwards that these institutions were consistently involved in the management of alcohol problems; Finnane (1981), for instance, estimates that at the end of the nineteenth century asylum administrators attributed about ten per cent of all admissions to intemperance. This is not to say that such admissions were encouraged or that public policy makers had developed a coherent ideological vision of alcoholism as a specific and treatable disease. While legal provision was made for the establishment of separate 'inebriate asylums', only one such institution was opened in Ireland and it functioned for just a short period.[5] Furthermore, the Intoxicating Liquor Commission of 1925 – the first major governmental committee to review alcohol issues in Ireland after self-government in 1922 – firmly rejected the idea that drinking problems should be conceptualised as diseases or that therapeutic institutions had a major role to play in societal management of drinking problems. Instead, the commission accepted public health arguments that the prevalence of drinking problems was a direct function of public access to alcohol and, on this basis, it recommended the retention of licensing and other control systems insofar as the electorate would tolerate such controls.[6]

Following the repeal of Prohibition in the USA in 1933, a number of stakeholders came together to promote the concept of alcoholism as a discrete disease, thought to be primarily attributable to the vulnerabilities of a small proportion of drinkers rather than to any inherent risk attaching to alcohol *per se*. The founding of Alcoholics Anonymous in 1935 was central to this process, but the growth of scientific interest in alcohol problems – particularly as represented in the opening of an alcohol research centre at Yale in 1939, and the establishment in 1944 of what was to become a National Council on Alcoholism (aimed at public education in this sphere) – were also key events in the American alcoholism movement of these years.[7] It was inevitable, given the cultural hegemony of the USA in the mid-twentieth century, that these ideas about alcoholism as a treatable disease would be diffused internationally and would, sooner or later, become influences on Irish policy makers.

For Irish policy makers in the period under study the two major options were to continue with a broad range of alcohol control measures, which could be seen as broadly health promotional in character, or alternatively to adopt the disease concept of alcoholism which was more narrowly concerned with curative services for problem drinkers. The material presented in this chapter will clearly indicate that until the early-1970s it was the latter option which was favoured: for more than a quarter of a century Irish health policy in relation to alcohol demonstrated a dominant concern with clinical concepts and practices, almost to the total exclusion of health promotional or preventive activities. The rest of this chapter will trace and describe the major events and institutions which made up this process, while at the same time seeking to identify the interest groups most actively involved either in advocating this medicalisation of drinking problems or in arguing against it. Given the key role which one could expect of the Department of Health in health policy formulation, and which is certainly envisaged by health promotion theorists, there will be a consistent focus on its activities in the alcohol sphere throughout the period considered here.

The World Health Organisation and the disease concept

Before proceeding with this account of developments in Irish alcohol policy, it is important to refer back to the international influence wielded in this sphere by the World Health Organisation (WHO) following its establishment in 1946. While the WHO generally displayed an interest in and commitment to what would later come to be referred to as 'health promotion', rather than an exclusive concern with the practice of medicine or with curative services, it deviated significantly from this policy approach in its handling of alcohol issues. The early WHO reports on alcoholism clearly reflect the influence of E.M. Jellinek, of the Yale Centre of Alcohol Studies, who worked as a consultant to the WHO from 1950 to 1955.[8] Understandably, Jellinek took with him to the WHO, through which he projected onto the international scene, all the preoccupations of the USA with what was sometimes referred to as the 'new scientific approach' to alcoholism. A 1952 publication of Jellinek's,[9] based on a survey of AA members, purported to depict the progression or natural history of alcoholism as a disease, suggesting that the disease process unfolded in an orderly, linear sequence, with each symptomatic stage inevitably building upon the previous stage. This chronological progression of alcoholism was graphically presented in a popular format, usually referred to as the 'Jellinek Chart'; a quarter of a century later the sociologist Robin Room suggested that 'this chart, particularly as adapted by Glatt (1970), is probably the most widely diffused artifact of the alcoholism movement's disease concept'.[10]

In overall terms, the impact of Jellinek on the WHO – and through this authoritative body on national health authorities – was to advance all the major tenets of the disease concept. Alcoholism was presented unambiguously to the world as a discrete disease which could be medically diagnosed, which had a predictable history and which deserved to be treated as other diseases were treated; while it was not claimed that its etiology was fully understood, it was generally suggested that alcoholism was primarily explicable in terms of individual deficit or predisposition, and it was argued that there was no relationship between societal levels of alcohol consumption and the incidence and prevalence of alcoholism. The Department of Health in Ireland was, therefore, subjected on this topic to a consistent and ostensibly authoritative stream of policy recommendations which pushed it in the direction of the disease concept favoured in the USA. In this context, the questions which must be asked are whether or how the Department of Health was influenced by the WHO. There was no obligation on the Department to accept WHO advice, but the manner in which it evolved its own approach to alcohol can be regarded as an example of its capacity to tackle complex health policy issues and to assess the value and relevance of external policy recommendations for the local Irish scene.

The Mental Treatment Act, 1945

The Mental Treatment Act, 1945 was the first mental health legislation to be enacted in Ireland in the period since self-government. It was for its time a progressive statute in that it provided for the voluntary admission of patients to psychiatric institutions and established a rudimentary set of safeguards against wrongful or unnecessary detention. It also provided a statutory basis for the creation of a range of outpatient psychiatric facilities, although such community-based services and facilities were not to be developed to any great extent for a further twenty years. In the context of this book, the Mental Treatment Act is important because it made specific provision for both the voluntary and compulsory admission to psychiatric hospital of 'addicts', this word clearly being intended to include those addicted to alcohol. It is perhaps helpful to cite in full the definition of an addict contained in the legislation. In this Act the word 'addict' means a person who –

(a) by reason of his addiction to drugs or intoxicants is either dangerous to himself or others or incapable of managing himself or of ordinary proper conduct, or

(b) by reason of his addiction to drugs, intoxicants or perverted conduct is in serious danger of mental disorder.[11]

In addition to some difficulties with the concept of 'ordinary proper conduct' which were raised during the legislative process and which will be discussed below, there is of course a fundamental difficulty with a definition of an addict which appears to regard the underlying concept of addiction as self-explanatory and in no need of definition. However, the importance of this inclusion of and reference to addicts in the Mental Treatment Act was that it provided a specific statutory basis for the expansion of alcoholism treatment within the Irish mental health system which was to take place in subsequent years. Critics of the scale of alcoholism treatment in Ireland, particularly the growth in in-patient care which took place from the late 1960s onwards, certainly were unhappy with this provision of the legislation, and it became increasingly likely that it would be omitted from new mental health legislation. Dermot Walsh, a psychiatrist who through his varied roles as clinician, epidemiologist and Inspector of Mental Hospitals exerted considerable influence on the Irish psychiatric care system for almost forty years, described this provision of the 1945 legislation and its consequences as he saw them in the following terms:

> The 'medicalisation' of alcohol problems continued at the same rate here as elsewhere and was codified by the provisions of the 1945 Mental Treatment Act which in addition to encouraging the voluntary admission of 'alcoholics' to psychiatric hospitals made provision for their compulsory admission as well. ... One consequence of this was that in line with increased consumption of alcohol, admission for this condition had become the most common cause of admission to psychiatric hospitals and units and by the mid-1970s constituted one-half of all male admissions and one-third of all admissions for both sexes.[12]

In view of these subsequent developments in the demands made by and resources allocated to alcoholism treatment in the Irish mental health system, it is important to consider in detail what the policy intent of the Minister for Health was in including this provision in the legislation. Was it the Minister's intent that the psychiatric services should adopt a more positive and welcoming attitude to alcoholism? Did this inclusion of addiction in the legislation signify a coherent and decisive policy shift by the Minister and his department towards the disease concept?

Based on a careful study of such documents as are available on the enactment of the Mental Treatment Act, 1945, the answer to these questions is generally negative. An obviously striking fact is that, although the legislation had been in preparation for many years, the addiction provisions were not in the Bill (Mental Treatment Bill, 1944) but were introduced as an amendment by the parliamentary secretary, Dr Ward, at the committee stage. One can speculate that this amendment would not have been introduced were it not for the intervention of the Irish Medical Association (IMA); the IMA had been generally positive in its response to the Mental Treatment Bill, but an editorial article in the January 1945 issue of its journal critically noted the absence of any reference to alcoholism in the proposed legislation:

There is no mention in the Bill of methods for the control and treatment of drug addicts and alcoholics. This is an important, and in itself, a very difficult question. It bristles with legal difficulties, apart altogether from the medical aspects of the conditions and, of course, any doctor be he a general practitioner or a psychiatrist, knows how urgent this matter is. Much suffering and misery is caused particularly by the chronic alcoholic who cannot be controlled and who cannot be fully treated under the present system.[13]

More conclusively, however, in introducing the definition of addiction into legislation the parliamentary secretary made it clear that it was not intended that this inclusion should have an immediate impact on the way in which general psychiatric services and facilities were administered. Dr Ward's basic contention was that at some future time it might be possible to set up a separate system of specialist addiction services and that, against this eventuality, some specific statutory provision must be made. Following a lengthy comment on the difficulty and complexity of alcohol and drug problems, he summarised his policy intent on this matter:

I should tell the House that, at this stage, we can only provide the necessary [legal] machinery, and that until such time as suitable institutions are available we cannot deal adequately with the problem that this amendment is intended to deal with. It will only be in case of urgency, or particular emergency, that addicts will be received in the ordinary institutions. In the course of time it is hoped that we may be able to provide special institutions ...[14]

It was suggested by one opposition deputy that the inclusion of the phrase 'ordinary proper conduct' in the text of the bill was unacceptably vague and that it would put great pressure on admitting psychiatrists, particularly where relatives were anxious to have troublesome drinkers locked up; generally, it was argued by a number of opposition deputies that this definition of an addict would prove problematic for the psychiatric service. Dr Ward, in a series of exchanges which became increasingly fractious, would only concede that these deputies made 'a good enough debating point'.[15] While it is conceivable that some of this debate was of a mischievous kind, aimed at annoying Dr Ward who was not noted for his tolerance or even temperament,[16] it will emerge later in this chapter and in Chapter Four, that there was serious substance to the reservations expressed by these opposition deputies.

It can safely be concluded, therefore, that the inclusion of the addiction provision in the Mental Treatment Act, 1945 did not represent a decisive and well thought-out policy shift towards the disease concept. The amendment represented, instead, an eleventh-hour decision to acknowledge this complex issue, largely on the basis that at some future time – when resources or technical developments permitted – alcoholism would be tackled more decisively in specialist settings. Dr Ward's attitude towards the treatment of alcoholics in the general psychiatric system may well have been the same as that which had traditionally prevailed – alcoholics were admitted to psychiatric institutions largely on sufferance – but, as circumstances changed, what proved to be important was not his rationale for this amendment but simply the fact that there was now an explicit statutory basis for this practice. Even though it was not Dr Ward's or his department's intention, as other forces and interest groups promoted the disease concept of alcoholism, the Mental Treatment Act appeared to support the view that the psychiatric hospital should become, in the phrase of Dermot Walsh,[17] the 'preferred locale' for dealing with alcohol-related problems in Ireland.

Alcoholics Anonymous in Ireland

In considering the introduction of the AA to Ireland and its impact upon Irish society, it should be remembered that AA neither was nor purported to be a scientific or technical innovation which might be guaranteed an uncomplicated diffusion throughout the developed world. Kurtz, the author of what could be deemed to be an officially approved history of AA, has described it as a social movement clearly rooted in the culture and society in which it originated: 'in a score of ways, Alcoholics Anonymous was at least by association as American as baseball, apple pie and the Fourth of July'.[18] There is no reason, therefore, to suppose that its establishment in Ireland was inevitable or straightforward, and in view of the centrality of spiritual themes in AA it is particularly important to consider how it was viewed by the Roman Catholic Church in Ireland.

The first AA meeting in Ireland, which is also reputed to have been the first AA meeting in Europe, took place in late 1946 when Conor F., home from the USA on holiday, met Richard P., an in-patient in St Patrick's Hospital. The meeting was facilitated by Dr Norman Moore, Medical Director of St Patrick's.[19]

Richard P., who was apparently a chronic alcoholic, immediately responded to AA, in the process persuading Dr Moore of the value of this new American approach to alcoholism treatment. By the time Conor F. returned to Philadelphia in early 1947, a small AA network had been established, based in the Country Shop, St Stephen's Green, Dublin.

The increase in membership of AA in Ireland, as can be seen in Table 2, was steady rather than meteoric; nonetheless, these figures show that AA filled a need for increasing numbers of Irish people over its first forty years here and so became well placed to be an influence not merely on individual alcoholics but also – whether or not this was part of its official agenda – on the wider society.

Table 2: Membership figures for AA in Ireland

Year	1946	1956	1966	1976	1986
Membership	45	1,100	2,250	5,750	9,000

Source: AA Souvenir Booklet, 1986; these figures refer to the thirty-two counties and given the loose membership structure of the Fellowship, must be regarded as approximations.

In its souvenir booklet, published in 1986 for the Fellowship's fortieth anniversary in Ireland, the struggle to keep AA going during its early years is described, and the following two imperatives for organisational survival discussed. Two things were evident from the start:

(a)   either the Catholic Church in Ireland was made an ally or AA in Ireland was sunk, and
(b)   either AA publicised itself in Dublin or it would perish of dry rot.[20]

The latter task was relatively easily accomplished since the Dublin papers were willing to publish letters, news stories and features concerning the Fellowship. Indeed, despite frequent Fellowship references to the stigma attaching to alcoholism and to the alleged distaste of 'respectable' society for anything to do with alcoholism, there is no evidence that the newspapers in Ireland were anything other than interested and encouraging. AA was treated neither with indifference nor hostility, and its basic ideological stance on alcoholism as a spiritual disease was generally presented in an uncritical way.

   The potential for conflict with the Roman Catholic Church is perhaps best understood through a study of the defensive way in which apologists for AA presented their case, but in essence there were two main issues which could have proved to be stumbling blocks. The first of these concerns the question of moral culpability: the Roman Catholic Church in Ireland, indeed the Church universally, might have interpreted AA's claim to the 'sick role' as being an invalid or dubious attempt to exonerate alcoholics from moral responsibility for their misbehaviour. As late as 1960, the theologian Fr Seán O'Riordan, a long-time defender and advocate of AA, felt it necessary to explain to a conference on *The Priest and Mental Health* that the compulsive nature of alcoholism meant that these excessive drinkers *wanted* to recover from their habit but *could* not:

   Modern psychology, however, throws a good deal of light on it. Such a craving is a 'compulsion' which cripples its victims alcoholically, as other compulsions cripple men in other spheres of human life. It operates to diminish, sometimes substantially diminish, his responsibility for his behaviour, and it is resistant to all direct attempts to counter it, even when these come from within the personality of the sufferer, in virtue of his rational and spiritual will.[21]

The second, and probably the more serious issue, concerns the spiritual nature of AA's programme. While it might appear that AA's insistence on spiritual values, on moral inventories and on the importance of having recourse to a Higher Power would be ideologically compatible with Roman Catholicism, the truth was that such an explicitly spiritual programme ran the risk of being seen as threatening to usurp the role of the Church in Ireland. AA had its roots in the Protestant evangelical tradition of the USA, and had been introduced to Dublin through what would have then been described as a 'Protestant' hospital, having failed to secure the support of a 'Catholic' hospital; this being the case, it seemed ripe for attack by the redoubtable Dr John Charles McQuaid, Roman Catholic Archbishop of Dublin at this time.[22] The new Fellowship was fortunate, therefore, to find an ally in Canon J.G. McGarry, Professor of Pastoral Theology at St Patrick's College, Maynooth, and editor of *The Furrow*, who throughout the 1950s allowed this influential publication to be used consistently in support of AA.

The first *Furrow* article on AA was written in 1952 by Fr Seán O'Riordan, consisting of a summary and discussion of a similar article in an American pastoral magazine. O'Riordan cited from this American article the proposition that: 'Alcoholics Anonymous insists more vigorously on the practice of Christian ascetics and the spiritual life than do priests of the Church of Christ'.[23] This was obviously dangerous stuff, where AA appeared to claim that help from the Higher Power, operating through its Fellowship, rivaled or outstripped the Roman Catholic Church which tended to see itself as the supreme channel of Divine Grace. In his 1960 conference paper to an audience of priests and medical doctors, O'Riordan was still dealing with this delicate theme:

> Some priests have been chary about invoking the help of this movement because of its undenominational character. Would not a similar movement but on specifically Catholic lines, they ask, be much better suited to our conditions and be more effective too, since then *all* the Church's sources of grace would be brought directly into play in helping the alcoholic back to sobriety and steady living?[24]

On a related theme, O'Riordan had argued in an early paper that: 'The organisation is not, of course, a secret society in any sense'.[25] This defence was necessary because AA, with its trappings of secrecy and anonymity, did evoke images of secret societies which – both of a religious and a political nature – were well-known in Ireland. If one applies the old sociological concepts of *in-group* and *out-group,* the convention of anonymity is understandable in the sense that, in societal terms, alcoholics perceived themselves to be an out-group – misunderstood, stigmatised and marginalised – who used their anonymity to protect themselves. However, having joined together in Fellowship, they obviously established their own in-group and, understandably perhaps, tended at times to emphasise the defining characteristics of alcoholics in positive terms rather than solely in terms of pathology. While it did not represent official AA teaching and may not always have been taken seriously by a majority of members, this positive depiction of themselves and their Fellowship could on occasion appear to outsiders like a form of inverted snobbery, almost as though alcoholics claimed to be superior to others and to belong to an exclusive club. This aspect of AA and the provocative self-image which some alcoholics cultivated was exemplified in yet another *Furrow* article published in 1953 by an author who simply signed himself 'a Victim':

> In conclusion I would like to emphasise that alcoholism is more often than not simply the result of heredity, environment or other untoward circumstances entirely outside the victim's volition. Men of the highest intellect and culture and with the most generous outlook fall the easiest victims to its insidious approach, their very sensitiveness to all that is false, unjust and anomolous in a topsy-turvy world rendering them all the more vulnerable ...[26]

In the main, however, AA managed its entry into Irish society with considerable skill, and with the support of Canon McGarry and the deft handling of potentially dangerous issues by Fr O'Riordan, avoided direct conflict with the Roman Catholic Church. In fact, its strength in Ireland is unusual, given that AA has generally not thrived in predominantly Roman Catholic cultures. A delegation of Irish AA members travelled to Rome in 1972 to commemorate the Fellowship's silver jubilee in Ireland, and while there had an audience with Pope Paul VI; one of the party later described this audience for *Furrow* readers, noting with surprise that the Pope, while welcoming, knew virtually nothing about AA![27]

In summarising this material in terms of its implications for health policy in Ireland, what is most important and bears repeating is that AA had absolutely nothing to say on the subject of prevention or health promotion. The AA programme was, as in its country of origin, entirely concerned with the recovery of individual alcoholics; recovery, of course, was seen as a life-long task of which total abstinence from alcohol was the *sine qua non.* By concentrating attention on a minority of 'diseased' drinkers AA contributed, albeit unintentionally, to a process of deflecting attention away from the wider context of drinking in Irish society.

The organisational principles of AA – as codified in its Twelve Traditions – specifically precluded it from involvement in outside debate or public controversy, which effectively meant that AA in Ireland did not contribute to policy debate or act as a lobbyist in relation to any aspect of national alcohol policy. By implication, however, because of its individualistic approach to etiology, AA called into question the value of control policies and favoured the provision of treatment facilities for individual alcoholics. In the USA, AA members – notably Marty Mann who was commonly referred to as the first woman to recover through AA – had circumvented the Fellowship ban on lobbying by doing so through another organisation, the National Council on Alcoholism. The creation of an Irish equivalent was obviously an option open to Irish AA members who wished to become involved in alcohol policy.

Liberalising the licensing laws

The licensing legislation which regulated the opening hours of Irish public houses had been quite restrictive since the founding of the State, particularly in relation to Sunday trading. In the mid-1940s, licensed premises in the four county boroughs of Dublin, Cork, Limerick and Waterford were allowed to do general trading between 1pm and 3pm (or to be precise 1.30 and 3pm in Dublin), and between 5pm and 7pm.[28] In rural areas, however, there was no general opening on Sundays, but *bona fide* trading was allowed between 1pm and 5pm (8pm in the summer). The *bona fide* system was a traditional arrangement which allowed genuine (hence the phrase *bona fide*) travellers to have access to licensed premises for refreshments at times when the general retailing of alcoholic beverages was not allowed. Being more than three miles (or in urban areas five miles) distant from one's usual residence made one a *bona fide* traveller, and by the 1940s this was being widely used by drinkers as a pretext for having longer drinking hours than were legally available in the local pub. As the motor car became a more common form of transport, the *bona fide* system obviously increased the dangers of road traffic accidents as drinkers were inclined to drive in groups to '*bona fide* houses', particularly those pubs on the outskirts of Dublin which specialised in this trade.

In 1948 and again in 1950 a Fianna Fáil backbench member of the Dail, Mr Martin Corry, unsuccessfully introduced private members' bills which would allow general Sunday opening throughout the country; his rationale on each of these occasions was that there was no longer any popular support for Sunday closing, that the law was being constantly flouted and that the Gardaí were increasingly unwilling to enforce it. Mr Corry's bills were defeated, not on public health grounds but by a more fundamentalist moral argument. In 1948, following a denunciation of the Corry bill by the Roman Catholic hierarchy, there was little political support for the idea that rural Ireland should be allowed to drink on Sundays and, in the course of a long and colourful speech in Dáil Éireann, Oliver Flanagan of Fine Gael asked the following questions:

> Does he desire to see a state of affairs prevail in this country whereby on the dark wintry Sundays in rural districts, the young boys and young men will, immediately they leave Mass, plunge their way into various public houses and remain there? ... Does he know that intemperance exists to a very large extent in this country at the moment? ... Does he know that champagne is cheaper today than it has been for a considerable time past, thanks to Fianna Fáil?[29]

Even in 1948, there must have been a certain amount of wry amusement at this image of the flower of Irish manhood crowding into bars and gorging itself on cheap champagne after Sunday Mass, but Deputy Flanagan's basic sentiments were apparently shared by a majority of Dáil Deputies and Deputy Corry's bill fell at its first hurdle. In 1950, the Roman Catholic hierarchy responded to the Corry private member's bill with even greater ferocity, citing Canon Law in support of its contention that any political activity directed towards generalised Sunday opening was sinful; as John Whyte put it, 'not only was the proposed legislation wrong, but even to make a case for it was wrong'.[30]

In 1956, however, the Minister for Justice appointed a Commission of Inquiry consisting of twenty-two people, chaired by the Master of the High Court and including representatives of the licensed trade, trades unions, Bord Fáilte, the Pioneer Total Abstinence Association and Dáil Éireann to review the licensing laws. Significantly, there was no health representative on this body, nor does there appear to have been any coherent health submission to the Commission, either by way of oral evidence or written documentation. Like its 1925 predecessor, this Commission insisted that popular support was essential for the successful enforcement of licensing legislation, and the advice which it received from representatives of the judiciary and the Garda Síochána – particularly in relation to Sunday trading – was that existing legislation was now so unpopular as to be virtually unenforceable. The Garda Commissioner had also supplied evidence to the Commission to the effect that drunkenness was no longer a serious problem in Ireland: 'In 1955, prosecutions for drunkenness totalled 3,782 as compared with 7,165 in 1925 and 45,670 in 1912'.[31] While the Commission could only speculate as to the causes of this improvement, it still expressed the view that extending the hours of opening of retail outlets would not have a negative impact on this trend.

What was specifically different from the 1925 Intoxicating Liquor Commission was the absence of a public health voice to articulate the view that alcohol, despite its cultural acceptability and economic significance, was a noxious agent for which control policies were legitimate, if not absolutely necessary. Instead, the tone of the Commission's 1957 report, and the subsequent parliamentary debate which led to the enactment of the Intoxicating Liquor Act, 1960, suggested that the policy environment was in a process of significant change. The idea that the State, in the interests of public health, public order or morality, might seek to control the drinking habits of its citizens was now coming to be seen as paternalistic and old-fashioned. While there was a minority report and a number of dissenting observations (none of which, it should be added, advocated anything approximating to a public health approach), the general tone of the main report was that the mature citizens of a modern democracy could not be denied a more flexible licensing code. The major recommendations, accordingly, were that the *bona fide* system should be abolished, that closing time on weekdays should be 11.30pm and that Sunday opening throughout the country should be from 12.30pm to 2.00pm and 5.00pm to 9.00pm.

Not only did the Pioneer representative sign the majority report but, subsequently, in the September 1957 issue of its monthly magazine, *The Pioneer*, a correspondent, writing under the pen-name Chaunticlere, vigorously defended the recommended changes, suggesting that the strongest opposition to them would come from publicans who had specialised in *bona fide* trading and from staff unions which would resist the longer opening hours. This correspondent was aware of the irony involved in a situation where a temperance activist was in favour of extended opening hours, in the face of opposition from some who were directly involved in retailing liquor: 'Again, many [Pioneers] may find themselves more than a little dismayed to be cast in the roll *[sic]* of the champions of liberality while the licensed trade act as the apostles of temperance'.[32]

This support of the Pioneers for the proposed liberalisation of the licensing laws did not however represent an official or consensus view of the Roman Catholic Church in Ireland, and shortly before the publication of the Intoxicating Liquor Bill, 1959, the Roman Catholic hierarchy issued a statement decrying the recommendations of the Commission. The central thesis of the hierarchy's brief statement was that:

> Increased facilities for obtaining intoxicating liquor by the extension of the general opening hours will inevitably lead to a greater extension of alcoholism which, in modern conditions, has most serious moral and social effects in the increase of delinquency and in widespread danger to life on the roads.[33]

The passage of this legislation through the Oireachtas was lengthy and all aspects of the proposed changes were debated exhaustively, but it became clear that the Government (a single-party Fianna Fáil Government) was determined to implement the major policy recommendations of the Commission. The Taoiseach, Seán Lemass, made generally placatory remarks apparently aimed at the bishops, but it was the Minister for Justice, Oscar Traynor, who dealt specifically with the bishops' contention that, if enacted, this legislation would lead to an increase in the incidence of alcoholism. The Minister reported that inquiries to the Department of Health had revealed that the annual number of patients treated for alcoholism in the country's mental hospitals was of the order of one fortieth of one per cent of the adult population. He went on:

> There have been suggestions that alcoholism – as distinct from drunkenness – is a serious problem in this country and that it is on the increase. If by alcoholism is meant addiction to alcohol, necessitating treatment in mental institutions, I think I can reassure the house that alcoholism is not a national problem. Alcoholism is a problem, of course, even if a few people only were suffering from this disease, for addiction to alcohol must be recognised for what it is, a disease that requires medical treatment for the rehabilitation of the alcoholic.[34]

In concluding this argument, Mr Traynor cited one of the Jellinek-inspired WHO reports in support of his contention that there was no significant association between *per capita* consumption of alcohol and the incidence of the disease of alcoholism. It is, of course, difficult to know how convinced the Minister for Justice was of the scientific validity of the disease concept, but it seems likely that having decided to ignore the advice of the bishops, he certainly appreciated its political value. The enactment of this liberalised licensing legislation presented the health sector with an opportunity to voice its opinion on the health implications of making alcohol more accessible to the populace, an opportunity which it had not been given through representation on the Commission in 1956 and 1957. It seems reasonable to infer that during the process of inter-departmental consultation, which is part of the wider legislative process, the Department of Health had simply accepted the WHO line on alcoholism as a disease and had transmitted these views to the Department of Justice. The disease concept put a scientific gloss on drinking problems, rendering obsolete moral and political arguments such as those of the Catholic bishops.

The most sustained, fundamentalist criticism of the Bill during its passage through the Dáil came once again from Deputy Oliver Flanagan of Fine Gael. However, in the context of the overall debate, his appeal on this occasion to his colleagues to reject the Bill and 'to stand over the teaching of the Catholic Bishops as Catholics in a Catholic Parliament'[35] was beginning to sound anachronistic and to fall on largely deaf ears. There was little opposition to the Intoxicating Liquor Bill in the Seanad, and one Senator in particular, Tomás Ó Maoláin, greeted it euphorically as symbolic of the new and modern Ireland which was thought to be emerging:

> This is the sixth decade of the twentieth century and this is a civilised community. We are no better and no worse perhaps than others but certainly we are as well-conducted as any. We are building up a modern progressive democracy. There is no reason why we should fear to get into line with other modern and progressive States which trust their people to be rational in using the liberal facilities they provide for drinking.[36]

The Intoxicating Liquor Act, 1960 was the first, and for a long time the only, instance of Irish legislative behaviour which ignored the advice of the Roman Catholic hierarchy. In enacting this relatively liberal licensing code, the Government obviously felt that the Irish public was so committed to this change that it could take the unprecedented risk of ignoring the bishops. The argument of the bishops was that, regardless of public opinion, it was morally and socially wrong to make alcohol more readily accessible; the duty of legislators, in the view of the hierarchy, was to retain and enforce the existing legislation, much as they would enforce unpopular finance legislation where failure to do so would result in social chaos. As previously stated, there was no public health voice raised in support of the bishops; on the contrary, the Minister for Justice could and did invoke the WHO to argue that the views of the hierarchy were unscientific and out-of-date.

The Irish National Council on Alcoholism

In 1964 the journalist Michael Viney published a series of articles on alcoholism in the *Irish Times,* which were later published in booklet form and were apparently well received by many people.[37] Viney's articles were thoroughly researched and well written, and by and large they reflected and promoted the disease concept of alcoholism. Although AA had by now established itself in Ireland on an apparently sound footing and although alcoholics continued to be admitted to the country's psychiatric hospitals, Viney was critical of what he saw as the lack of a sustained and coherent national response to this problem, and recommended the establishment of a 'National Council on Alcoholism', comparable to that which existed in Britain and the USA. He suggested that an attempt to establish such a council had failed some years previously because 'even supposedly intelligent and highly-educated men were afraid of the stigma they thought would attach to such patronage'.[38] In 1966, however, following a visit to Ireland by Marty Mann of the American National Council on Alcoholism, the Irish National Council on Alcoholism (INCA) was set up in Dublin.

Although INCA was later to portray itself as being representative of 'an influential cross-section of Irish professional and business personalities',[39] it would appear that the initiative for its establishment came from a somewhat narrower range of interests, primarily representing psychiatrists in the private sector and AA members. One of these private sector psychiatrists, Dr John Cooney of St Patrick's Hospital, acknowledged this later when, in a 1980 publication, he wrote that he took 'some pride in the fact that the Irish National Council on Alcoholism was set up in 1966 through the initiative of a few psychiatrists'. In fact, four of the seven subscribers to the organisation's Memorandum of Association were private sector psychiatrists, while two, although they did not publicly declare themselves as such, were prominent members of AA.[40] There is no evidence that the Department of Health played any role in the establishment of INCA and, as will be discussed later in this chapter, statutory health funding for INCA remained low until 1973.

The aims of INCA were set out in detailed legalese in its Memorandum and Articles of Association, but, in summary, it can be said that it had one dominant aim, which was to promote the disease concept of alcoholism at the level of public awareness, the level of treatment service provision and the level of scientific research. Like its American counterpart, INCA deliberately avoided any criticism of alcohol or any suggestion that, in public health terms, alcohol was a dangerous substance; its strict neutrality on this issue was exemplified in the manner in which its Articles of Association, having set out its main aims, enjoined the organisation to 'pursue these objects without making any judgement upon the consumption of alcohol *per se*'.[41] Thus there was to be no advice to the public about moderate drinking, and no focus in its publicity on questions of toxicity or addictiveness. Instead, INCA intended to follow the line laid down by its American progenitor by emphasising the primacy of individual predisposition in the etiology of alcoholism. In the sphere of practical politics this neutrality also meant that INCA had no qualms about seeking or accepting financial support from the drinks industry, and the organisation's First Annual Report coyly acknowledged the importance for its survival of 'a substantial donation from a world-famous Brewery in Dublin'.[42]

The influence of AA on INCA was not confined to the presence of two members of AA on the council: the first Executive Director of INCA was Richard Perceval, none other than Richard P. who as the first Irish-based member of AA had done so much to advance the cause of AA in Ireland.

Following the precedent of Marty Mann in the USA, Mr Perceval – who had been involved between 1962 and 1966 with the establishment of a British Council on Alcoholism – had now set aside his anonymity to engage in the kind of political lobbying which was impossible under the aegis of AA. The views expressed by Mr Perceval were similar to those to be found in the American alcoholism scene; although he railed against what he saw as the lack of understanding of alcoholism and the associated stigma, it is difficult in retrospect to find evidence for the existence of any significant or orchestrated opposition to the disease concept in Ireland at this time. A 1970 pamphlet of Perceval's, which contained the contention that 'the ideal climate of opinion is one in which dependence upon alcohol is openly regarded as something just as real, just as serious as tuberculosis – but no more culpable' was in fact published by Veritas, the main publishing outlet for the Catholic Church in Ireland, which had previously been known as the Catholic Truth Society of Ireland.

Given INCA's neutrality on the issue of alcohol and its preoccupation with treatment for individual alcoholics, it is not surprising to find that Perceval's views on primary prevention were somewhat limited. He took it for granted that there was no meaningful connection of a causal kind between alcohol and alcoholism, and therefore saw little sense in public health messages which might advocate safe or moderate drinking. In an article published in *The Pioneer* at around the time that INCA was established, he wrote:

> Prevention in its true sense is impossible, as we do not know the cause. But *secondary* prevention or the reduction of damage is feasible by education, by information and by understanding. It is possible to produce a climate of opinion in which anyone who has the primary symptoms of alcoholism will feel it is a duty – *not* a disgrace – to do something about it.[43]

Just as Marty Mann had made exaggerated claims for the scientific status of the views which she promoted through her organisation in New York (claims which were frequently disputed by members of the scientific community), so too did Richard Perceval present his own views as being objectively and scientifically beyond dispute, while those who disagreed with him were portrayed as misguided or moralistic. Although INCA established an advisory and referral service at its Dublin headquarters, most of its activities during its early years were of a promotional or educational type; this mainly consisted of giving or arranging public talks on the disease concept, as well as using the media to disseminate its message. Whatever about the content of this message, it has to be concluded that, as INCA's first Director, Richard Perceval was an energetic and apparently effective lobbyist.

As already noted, the Department of Health played no role in the establishment of INCA; indeed INCA remained a voluntary body all through the twenty-two years of its existence, even after it began to be completely funded by the regional health boards in 1973. The attitude of the Department of Health towards INCA was generally positive and encouraging, but this did not extend as far as making any financial commitment to its support; in fact at the time of its establishment, the Minister for Health, Seán Flanagan, expressed the hope that INCA would receive whatever funding it required from industrial and business concerns.[44] The brief comments on INCA which are to be found in the 1966 Report of the *Commission of Inquiry on Mental Illness* (to which, tacitly at least, the Department of Health gave its approval) suggest that the Department understood and approved of INCA's philosophy and action plan. There was one subtle but important point, however, which suggested that the Commission did not fully appreciate what INCA's (or at least Perceval's) position was: this was in relation to prevention, where the Commission expected that 'this Council will serve an important preventive and advisory function by spreading knowledge on the dangers of excessive and indiscriminate drinking'.[45] As is clear from the earlier discussion of his views, Perceval regarded alcoholics as hapless victims of a mysterious ailment rather than as people who indulged in excessive or indiscriminate drinking, and he showed no inclination to provide education along 'sensible drinking' lines for the Irish public.

INCA was, as has been made clear, a council on 'alcoholism' rather than a council on 'alcohol'. At least in its early years, it was powerfully influenced by AA and this influence, allied to that of psychiatry, conspired to advance the cause of treatment almost to the total exclusion of prevention. The Department of Health played no role in setting up INCA, neither did it overwhelm INCA with support in its early years; it gradually moved beyond the stage of merely offering moral support to a time (which will be discussed in Chapter Three) where it provided full financial support for the organisation. Just as it had seen no health implications to the liberalising of the licensing laws, so too did the Department of Health appear to have identified nothing problematic in this tendency of INCA's to focus solely on treatment and to exonerate alcohol of any causal responsibility for alcohol-related problems.

Treatment services for alcoholics

The material covered in this chapter generally indicates that for a quarter of a century after World War II a range of influences and interests in Ireland shifted public policy towards the disease concept of alcoholism, away from its previous alcohol control ethos. For the health care system in Ireland the major implication of this shift was the expectation, if not the demand, that there would be an expansion of treatment and rehabilitation services for alcoholics; furthermore, there was an expectation that in attitudinal terms alcoholism would become a 'respectable' disease and that any moralism or residual stigma would be eliminated from within the health care system. The pace of this policy change was slow and gradual, and one cannot identify any dramatic turning point. There are, however, two further events, the establishment of the Voluntary Health Insurance (VHI) Board in 1957 and the publication (already alluded to) of the *Report of the Commission of Inquiry on Mental Illness* in 1966, which deserve some comment before concluding this account of the institutionalisation of the disease concept within Irish health policy.

The Voluntary Health Insurance Board was established by statute in 1957; its aim was to allow people in the middle and upper income groups, who were not eligible or had only limited eligibility for the means-tested public health service, to insure themselves and their dependants against the high costs of hospital treatment and maintenance. VHI was a state-sponsored, non-profit organisation which was given a monopoly on the sale of health insurance in Ireland, a monopoly which endured until the mid-1990s when it was withdrawn as part of Ireland's integration into the European Community. The VHI scheme was made additionally attractive to subscribers by the tax relief on insurance premiums allowed by the Minister for Finance, and it proved from the outset to be a viable and popular system.

One unanticipated consequence of this development was that middle-class alcoholics, who had previously been reluctant to seek treatment in the spartan public mental hospitals, were now a good deal more willing – courtesy of their VHI cover – to agree to admission to the relatively salubrious private hospitals. These hospitals were rooted in a religious and philanthropic tradition, rather than in the 'for-profit' ethos of modern American health-care institutions; nonetheless, it is scarcely a coincidence that once a funding system was set in place which guaranteed a flow of alcoholic patients through their institutions, these hospitals began to play a much more vocal role in advocating the disease concept. There were obvious financial incentives for hospitals to develop alcoholism treatment programmes for these patients, who were available in constant numbers, who made relatively little demands of the nursing and medical system once detoxified, and whose bills – thanks to VHI – were sure to be paid.

The question of differences of attitude and practice in relation to alcoholism treatment between psychiatrists in private hospitals and their colleagues in the public sector will be considered more explicitly in

Chapter Three. However, during the period 1945-1972, which is dealt with in the present chapter, there was no evidence of conflict between these two groups. Instead, the position was, as exemplified in the INCA situation, that psychiatrists from the private sector campaigned without equivocation – and, it must be said, without being critically challenged – for the universal acceptance of the disease concept. A particularly good example of such advocacy is to be found in a 1963 paper, addressed primarily to general medical practitioners, by Dr John Cooney of St Patrick's Hospital, Dublin. The lead role played by the private hospitals is suggested by the figures cited by Dr Cooney: 'In 1960, 532 alcoholics were treated in private mental hospitals in Ireland, while 107 were that year admitted to district mental hospitals.' He also told his readers that:

> If one is to treat alcoholism successfully whether in hospital or in general practice one must feel as well as believe that the alcoholic is ill and suffering from a disease just as surely as a diabetic is suffering from his excess blood sugar ... [B]y their acceptance of the disease concept of alcoholism they [doctors] can influence public opinion and help bring about an attitude whereby the alcoholic is regarded not as a moral degenerate but as a sick man ...[46]

The clearest and most unequivocal public policy acceptance of the disease concept, which must surely have been pleasing to psychiatrists from the private sector, to members of AA and to the newly established INCA, was contained in the *Report of the Commission of Inquiry on Mental Illness*. This Commission was established by the Minister for Health in 1961 to review and make recommendations on the functioning of the country's mental health services and legislation; it reported in 1966, generally recommending a move towards community rather than residential services. On the question of alcoholism, the Commission fully endorsed the disease concept, prefacing its discussion and recommendations by the summary statement: 'Alcoholism is a disease and is regarded by the World Health Organisation as a major health problem'.[47] The recommendations referred both to community and residential treatment facilities; in the former case it was suggested that general practitioners, in consultation with consultant psychiatrists, could offer valuable treatment to alcoholic patients, while in the latter it was suggested that specialist in-patient units should be created within the public psychiatric system to complement the work being done in this field by the private hospitals. The Commission concluded that specialist staff were needed to cater for alcoholics; but '[i]n view of this fact and of the relatively small number of alcoholics needing residential treatment the Commission considers that alcoholic units in three or four regional centres would meet the country's needs'.[48]

The recommendation that GPs should be more involved in the treatment of alcoholics largely represented a pious aspiration and no coherent strategy was ever devised to make this a reality; there is evidence, it must be said, that the Irish situation in this regard is broadly similar to that which prevails elsewhere.[49] However, the conclusion that Ireland had only a small number of alcoholics needing residential treatment and that four regional units would suffice in the public health sector must surely be regarded as a policy miscalculation of quite heroic proportions. The logic underlying this policy perspective was similar to that invoked during the debate on the Intoxicating Liquor Bill, 1959: it was assumed that the incidence of alcoholism was static and, accordingly, that there was no reason to believe that increased public access to alcohol or increased consumption rates would lead to increased demands for treatment and rehabilitation. Statistical data documenting the dramatic increase in the treated prevalence of alcoholism from the late 1960s onwards will be presented in Chapter Three; suffice it to say here that within five years of the Commission's report the number of alcoholism admissions to Irish psychiatric hospitals and units had doubled, and within ten years almost one in four admissions to the in-patient mental health system had a primary diagnosis of alcoholism. The prospect of confining such admissions to four regional alcohol units quickly disappeared; the reality was that alcoholism treatment made big demands on all forms of in-patient care – on private psychiatric hospitals, on health board psychiatric hospitals and on the emerging general hospital psychiatric units.

Conclusion

It could be surmised that the alcohol control policies which had evolved in Ireland from the second half of the nineteenth century, and which had found particularly clear expression in the Intoxicating Liquor Commission 1925, would not withstand the challenge of the American disease concept unless they were periodically restated and their value and legitimacy defended. The material discussed in the present chapter clearly demonstrates that no such defence or restatement of the alcohol control perspective was made in Ireland in the quarter of a century following World War II. Furthermore, it has emerged that none of the main interest groups or institutions which might have taken exception to the disease concept did, in fact, do so.

On the contrary, all the major players in this arena gave a general, if somewhat gradual, welcome to the 'new scientific approach' to drinking problems. The Roman Catholic Church objected only to the extension of the opening hours of pubs, and in particular to Sunday opening, but was otherwise open to and accepting of the various ideological and institutional strands of the disease concept. Similarly, the criminal justice system supported the new policy line, as did treatment professionals in the mental health field – particularly following the establishment of VHI.

There is no evidence, however, that the Department of Health played a key role in either initiating or co-ordinating this policy process. To use the language of health promotion, the Department of Health demonstrated no appreciation of 'healthy public policy': it did not anticipate that making alcohol more accessible would ultimately have negative health consequences or see that that there were legitimate health arguments to be made against the new licensing scheme. Instead, it appeared to stand back from events, merely allowing things to happen for much of the period looked at in this chapter. The Department was obviously aware of and influenced by the WHO's commitment to the disease concept, as exemplified by its advice to the Minister for Justice at the time the Intoxicating Liquor Bill, 1959 was being debated. However, it was only when a considerable momentum had gathered in favour of the disease concept that the Department of Health gave a clear and explicit commitment to that concept in 1966, through its acceptance of the Report of the Commission of Inquiry on Mental Illness.

The policy-making process was not, therefore, of the rational-comprehensive variety: No formal policy analysis took place to clarify what cultural values were involved in this sphere, nor were policy objectives identified and then matched with the means likely to lead to their achievement. Instead, the policy process appears to fit the classic incremental pattern described by Lindblom. Means and ends are not clearly distinguished in this process of 'partisan mutual adjustment', where the test of a good policy is not that it conforms to agreed values or achieves identified objectives, but rather that it secures the agreement of as many as possible of the various interests involved. The great strength of the disease concept, in policy terms, was that it appeared to please everybody; from the drinks industry, through the drinking public, to those involved in alcoholism treatment there was consensus as to the value and validity of this perspective.

However, the disease concept of alcoholism was antithetical to practically every tenet of the health promotion model outlined in Chapter One. At the level of healthy public policy, as this is understood within the health promotion paradigm, the disease concept implied that multisectoral co-operation in legislative and general policy terms was neither necessary nor useful. Similarly, the disease concept saw no value in such health promotion ideas as *lifestyle* or *environment*. Drinking lifestyles were irrelevant within a biomedical perspective which suggested that alcoholics were a minority, born with a predisposition to this disease; if you were unfortunate enough to be born with this predisposition, then even low alcohol consumption invariably triggered the disease process, while the majority not so afflicted could more or less drink with impunity. Finally, the idea of strengthening community action as a means of promoting health also had little chance of being operationalised, although AA, a self-help movement for sufferers of this disease, gained ever-increasing respect and credibility for its own version of the disease concept. AA was certainly a 'bottom-up' policy initiative, and one which was to be enormously influential in the growth of other self-help health movements, but it had no interest in health promotion and implicitly reinforced the view that what was important was the provision of treatment facilities.

Even by the time the Commission of Inquiry on Mental Illness was giving its approval to the disease concept and INCA was being established to lobby for this viewpoint, there were indications that some of its most basic tenets might be flawed. Perhaps the most critical indicator was the increase in the treated incidence and prevalence of alcoholism, which raised the question of whether there might not be a causal connection between these increased demands on the health service and increased societal levels of alcohol consumption.

NOTES

1. The alcohol publications of SSISI between 1849 and 1858 have been summarised and commented upon in a recent SSISI paper: D. McCoy, *Issues for Irish Alcohol Policy: A Historical Perspective with Some Lessons for the Future.* (Paper read before the Statistical and Social Inquiry Society of Ireland, 24 October, 1991).

2. For a comprehensive history of nineteenth-century temperance in Ireland, see E. Malcolm, *Ireland Sober, Ireland Free: Drink and Temperance in Nineteenth Century Ireland.* (Dublin: Gill and Macmillan, 1986); for a history of the Roman Catholic 'Pioneer' movement see D. Ferriter, *A Nation of Extremes: The Pioneers in Twentieth-Century Ireland.* (Dublin: Irish Academic Press, 1999).

3. H.G. Levine, 'Temperance Cultures: concern about alcohol problems in Nordic and English-speaking cultures', in M. Lader, G. Edwards, and D.C. Drummond (eds), *The Nature of Alcohol and Drug Related Problems.* (Oxford University Press, 1992), pp 15-36.

4. M. Finnane, *Insanity and the Insane in Post-Famine Ireland.* (London: Croom Helm, 1981); J. Robins, *Fools and Mad.* (Dublin: Institute of Public Administration, 1986); J. Reynolds, *Grangegorman: Psychiatric Care in Dublin since 1815.* (Dublin: Institute of Public Administration, 1992).

5. B. Smith, 'Ireland's Ennis Inebriates Reformatory: a 19th century example of failed institutional reform', *Federal Probation* (March 1989), pp 53-64.

6. *Report of the Intoxicating Liquor Commission.* (Dublin: Stationery Office, 1925).

7.   E. Kurtz, *Not God: A History of Alcoholics Anonymous.* (Center City, Minnesota: Hazelden, 1991); E.M. Jellinek, *The Disease Concept of Alcoholism.* (New Haven: Hillhouse Press, 1960).

8.   For a brief discussion of Jellinek's work and influence at WHO see Chapter Twelve of K. Bruun, L. Pan and I. Rexed, *The Gentleman's Club: International Control of Drugs and Alcohol* (University of Chicago Press, 1975). For a more detailed study of Jellinek and his influence, see P. Page, 'E. M. Jellinek and the evolution of alcohol studies: a critical essay', *Addiction,* 92 (1997), pp 1619-1637.

9.   E. M. Jellinek, 'Phases of Alcohol Addiction', *Quarterly Journal of Studies on Alcohol, 13* (1952), pp 673-684.

10. R. Room, *Governing Images of Alcohol and Drug Problems.* (PhD Dissertation, University of California, Berkely, 1978), p.55.

11. Mental Treatment Act, 1945, Section 3.

12. D. Walsh, 'Alcohol and Alcohol Problems Research 15 – Ireland', *British Journal of Addiction, 82* (1987), pp 747-748.

13. 'Mental Treatment Bill, 1944' (Editorial Article), *Journal of the Medical Association of Éire,* 16 (1945), p.8.

14. *Dáil Debates* (Vol. 96), Column 1009.

15. Ibid, Column 1012.

16. See R. Barrington, *Health, Medicine and Politics in Ireland 1900-1970 .* (Dublin: Institute of Public Administration, 1987), pp 168-175.

17. D. Walsh, 'Alcohol and Ireland', *British Journal of Addiction,* 82 (1987), p.119.

18. E. Kurtz, *Not God: A History of Alcoholics Anonymous.* (Expanded Edition). (Center City, Minnesota: Hazelden, 1991), p.164.

19. The most authoritative source on the establishment of AA in Ireland used here is: *Alcoholics Anonymous in Ireland 1946-1986: A souvenir booklet to commemorate forty years of AA in Ireland.* (Dublin: AA General Service Conference of Ireland, 1986). Another important source was: Anthony Jordan, *Alcoholics Anonymous in Ireland* (M.Litt. Thesis, Trinity College Dublin, 2000).

20. *Alcoholics Anonymous in Ireland 1946-1986.* (This 16-page booklet cited above does not have its pages numbered).

21. S. O'Riordan, 'Alcoholism' in E.F. O'Doherty and S.D. McGrath (eds), *The Priest and Mental Health* (Dublin: Clonmore and Reynolds, 1962), p.151.

22. For a detailed description of Dr McQuaid and his controlling approach to health and social services see J. Cooney, *John Charles McQuaid: Ruler of Catholic Ireland.* (Dublin: O'Brien Press, 1999).

23. S. O'Riordan, *The Furrow* (January 1952), p.36.

24. S. O'Riordan, 'Alcoholism' in E.F. O'Doherty and S.D. McGrath, op.cit., p.151.

25. S. O'Riordan, *The Furrow* (May 1952), p.205.

26. 'A Victim', *The Furrow* (March 1953), p.146.

27. 'A Dublin Member of AA', 'Vatican and Alcoholics Anonymous' in 'News and Views', *The Furrow* (March 1972), p.182.

28. Factual data on pub opening hours are drawn from: *Reports of the Commission of Inquiry into the Laws relating to the Sale and Supply of Intoxicating Liquor 1957.* (Dublin: Stationery Office, 1957).

29. *Dáil Debates* (Vol.113), Columns 50-51.

30. J.H. Whyte, *Church and State in Modern Ireland, 1923-1979* (Second Edition). (Dublin: Gill and Macmillan, 1980), p.178.

31. *Reports of the Commission of Inquiry into the Laws relating to the Sale and Supply of Intoxicating Liquor 1957,* cit.sup., p.5.

32. 'Chaunticlere Discusses the Controversy about the Liquor Laws', *The Pioneer* (September 1957), pp 18-19.

33. *Statement of the Irish Bishops on the Intoxicating Laws issued at their June 1959 meeting at Maynooth, The Furrow* (August 1959), p.553.

34. *Dáil Debates* (Vol. 177), Column 948.

35. *Dáil Debates* (Vol. 180), Column 1029.

36. *Seanad Debates* (Vol. 52), Column 1601.

37. M. Viney, *Alcoholism in Ireland: An Inquiry.* (This is an undated reprint of the Michael Viney articles published by the *Irish Times,* apparently in 1964.)

38. M. Viney, op.cit., p.49.

39. *Report to the Minister for Health by the Irish National Council on Alcoholism* (January 1973), p.23.

40. *Memorandum and Articles of Association of the Irish National Council on Alcoholism, 1966.* The four psychiatrists were: Drs Moore and Cooney from St Patrick's Hospital, Dublin, and Drs McGrath and McCarthy from St John of God's Hospital, Dublin. Another subscriber, Sackville O'Connor Mallins, who was described as a retired army officer, was arguably the best-known of all the early AA organisers in Ireland, and it would appear that Aiden MacSweeney (described as a chemist) was also an AA member.

41. *Memorandum and Articles of Association of the Irish National Council on Alcoholism, 1966,* article 2(e).

42. *Irish National Council on Alcoholism, Annual Report February 1967 – February 1968.*

43. R. Perceval, 'Lack of Understanding', *The Pioneer* (July /August 1966), p.25.

44. *Irish Times* (17 November, 1966).

45. *Report of the Commission of Inquiry on Mental Illness.* (Dublin: Stationery Office, 1966), pp 82-83.

46. Ibid, pp 54-56.

47. *Report of the Commission of Inquiry on Mental Illness,* cit.sup., p.77.

48. Ibid, p. 82.

49. One of the most influential studies on the difficulties of developing a 'therapeutic commitment' to alcoholism amongst GPs and other primary care workers is: S. Shaw, A. Cartwright, T. Spratley and J. Harwin, *Responding to Drinking Problems.* (London: Croom Helm, 1978).

    A small-scale study of Irish GPs during 1993/94 revealed low therapeutic commitment to such clients – J. Connolly, *Doctors and Drinkers* (MEd thesis, St Patrick's College, Maynooth, 1994).

3

Conflicting Paradigms: The Disease Concept and the Public Health Perspective on Alcohol in Ireland 1973-1988

Introduction

If the period 1945-1972 was characterised by an emerging consensus concerning the scientific validity and political acceptability of the disease concept of alcoholism in Ireland, then the period 1973-1988, which is the subject of the present chapter, may be characterised as one of conflict. This conflict was between the disease concept and what came to be known as the *public health perspective* on alcohol; the latter perspective, which was articulated internationally from the mid-1970s onwards, conformed in remarkable detail to the wider health promotion paradigm which was also being developed at this time. Tables 3 and 4 are presented here to provide a context for the account of the public health perspective which is to follow and to demonstrate its relevance to the Irish policy scene. Essentially, what these tables indicate is that in the period when the disease concept of alcoholism was most influential there were major increases in alcohol consumption and that, contrary to expectations, increased consumption was related to an increased prevalence of problems (measured in this instance by just one indicator, psychiatric hospital admissions for alcoholism). The recognition of similar relationships between increased consumption levels and increases in prevalence in a range of alcohol-related problems internationally contributed to a radical revision of all the central tenets of the disease concept, and to the emergence of a public health approach emphasising the value of environmental policies of an alcohol control or regulatory nature.

The task facing those who advocated the public health perspective was obviously formidable coming, as it did, in the immediate aftermath of the popular acceptance of the disease concept. For policy makers and for the general public there was understandable confusion that, having been so recently persuaded of the scientific nature of the disease concept, they were now being asked – again for ostensibly scientific reasons – to abandon it and replace it with a diametrically different policy.

Table 3: Annual consumption of alcohol per head of population in Ireland (aged 15 and over) in litres of pure alcohol

Year	Total
1960	4.88
1961	5.36
1962	5.30
1963	5.50
1964	5.78
1965	5.87
1966	5.89
1967	6.01
1968	6.37
1969	6.91
1970	7.26
1971	7.68
1972	8.20
1973	8.88
1974	9.28
1975	9.22
1976	8.99
1977	9.20
1978	9.78
1979	9.97
1980	9.56
1981	9.02
1982	8.78
1983	7.97
1984	8.13
1985	8.56
1986	8.40
1987	8.12
1988	8.42
1989	8.65
1990	9.03
1991	9.12

Sources: CSO *Statistical Abstract,* various issues, Revenue Commissioners *Annual Report,* various years

The emergence of the public health perspective internationally

Despite the general consensus which marked the evolution of the disease concept in post-Prohibition America, social scientists had periodically expressed reservations about both the logic and the social desirability of this development. This sceptical approach to the disease concept was

Table 4: Alcohol-related admissions as a proportion of all admissions to Irish psychiatric hospitals and units for selected years

Year	All admissions	Alcohol admissions	Percentage of all admissions
1958	11,231	644	5.7
1965	15,350	1,638	10.7
1972	22,964	4,143	18.0
1979	27,358	7,158	26.2
1986	29,392	7,132	24.3
1993	27,005	5,718	21.2
1995	26,440	5,262	19.9

Sources: Report of the Inspector of Mental Hospitals for 1958, and *Annual Activities Reports* of the Medico-Social Research Board and Health Research Board

maintained as a central feature of the involvement of social scientists in the burgeoning alcohol research field in the USA and internationally. At the heart of this scepticism was the consistently expressed view that the promotion of the disease concept was more accurately to be thought of as a social movement than as the application of new scientific knowledge. One American sociologist, Seeley, in what proved to be a remarkably prescient critique published in 1962, argued as follows:

> As far as public communication is concerned, however, I think the bare statement that 'alcoholism is a disease' is most misleading, since (a) it links up with a much-too-narrow concept of 'disease' in the public mind, and (b) it conceals what is essential – that is, that a step in public policy is being *recommended,* not a scientific discovery announced. It would seem to me infinitely preferable to say, 'It is best to look on alcoholism as a disease because ...' and to enumerate reasons. This would both take the public into our confidence (and hence really educate) and permit withdrawal of the recommendation if it seemed wiser at a later date. The latter ought to be much easier and more comprehensible than a first announcement of a seeming scientific fact and its later contradiction with no new evidence.[1]

Such criticisms of the disease concept by social scientists were not, however, confined to America but were taken up at international level. A 1969 paper by Christie and Bruun, two Scandinavian sociologists with a particular interest in alcohol studies, argued trenchantly that this insistence that 'alcoholism is sickness' was acceptable and popular not despite but *because* of its vagueness and logical inconsistency; they described the disease concept, and related WHO ideas about illicit drugs, as 'big fat words' the function of which was to act as 'grease in the social machinery'.[2] In other words, Christie and Bruun rejected the idea that there was any technical or scientific base to the disease concept, and saw it instead as a pseudoscientific construct which allowed society to ignore the value and policy dilemmas inherent in this area. Where earlier generations had been accustomed to lively debate and controversy between 'wets' and 'drys', contemporary citizens of western democracies were being persuaded (according to Christie and Bruun) that science had made such debate redundant. The style of policy making favoured by these two sociologists was the rational comprehensive style in which value judgements could be clearly differentiated from scientific or technical developments; should this ever be achieved, it would bring 'conceptual refinement' to alcohol policy making, in the process 'giving to the experts what belongs to them, and to us all the decision on ethics which belongs to all of us'.[3]

In addition to these and other theoretical papers which predicted many negative social consequences stemming from an uncritical acceptance of the disease concept, empirical research also called into question some of its basic tenets. The success of the alcoholism movement in the USA had attracted substantial research funding; paradoxically, much of the empirical research undertaken with this financial support then contributed to the debunking of the alcoholism movement which had already been going on at a theoretical level.

Of major importance in this regard was the survey research carried out at the University of California, Berkeley, into the drinking habits of random samples of the population. Cahalan (1970) and Cahalan and Room (1974) found that drinking problems did not follow the progressive pattern described by Jellinek and members of AA. Instead, their longitudinal study showed that half of those drinkers identified in their base-line research as having an alcohol-related problem were drinking in a non-problematic way at three-year follow-up. They also found, however, that the proportion of problem drinkers remained the same, because those drinkers who moved from problem drinking to non-problem drinking were replaced by other drinkers moving in the opposite direction.[4]

The net effect of this research was to challenge the belief implicit in the disease concept that alcoholism progressed inevitably and inexorably unless the alcoholic became totally abstinent, and also to challenge the 'two population theory' – the view that alcoholism was a discrete disease so that drinkers could be categorically divided into 'alcoholics' and 'social drinkers'. Further blows to the scientific integrity of the disease concept resulted from continued reporting of moderate or controlled drinking among diagnosed and treated alcoholics who, according to the disease concept, ought to have quickly deteriorated, ultimately reaching the legendary 'rock bottom' at the lower end of the Jellinek Chart.

Predictably, research findings of this nature led to a radical questioning of the validity and utility of the disease concept, with its view of alcoholism as a discrete unitary disorder, as an explanatory device for what was now coming to be seen as a broad spectrum of problems. It was increasingly suggested that alcohol-related problems were multi-dimensional, involving physiological, psychological and behavioural elements, and that such problems did not necessarily involve *dependence* or alcoholism. The publication of a WHO report *Alcohol-Related Disabilities* in 1977 signalled a decisive move by that body away from its previous promotion of the disease concept. An editorial in *The Lancet* which discussed this report wondered whether its real message was that 'the hunt for a definition of alcoholism should be abandoned as the pursuit of what was never more than an imaginary animal', but concluded that the WHO could not abandon 'the reality of addiction to alcohol'.[5] Ultimately, the WHO adopted a classificatory system which saw alcohol problems as falling into one of two categories: *alcohol dependence* or *alcohol-related problems*. There were criticisms of the concept of alcohol dependence (or the alcohol dependence syndrome, as it was commonly referred to) by some social scientists, who regarded it as little more than a semantic change from alcoholism and as providing a spurious legitimation for the continuing pre-eminence of the medical profession in the field of alcohol problems. Nonetheless, this dualistic classification of drinking problems has remained within the WHO's *International Classification of Diseases* since 1979.

In the evolution of alternatives to the disease concept, another major landmark was the publication in 1975 of a collaborative study, *Alcohol Control Policies in Public Health Perspective*, by the Finnish Foundation for Alcohol Studies, in conjunction with WHO. This report argued that aggregate levels of alcohol consumption were among the best predictors of a society's incidence and prevalence of alcohol-related problems; in other words, it marked a return to a 'dry' policy perspective with its suggestion that the best way to reduce the incidence of such problems was through the limitation of consumption through various control measures. The WHO in an Expert Committee Report on *Problems Related to Alcohol Consumption* (1980) definitively confirmed this policy shift when it recommended that Member States should adopt alcohol control policies – principally through fiscal measures aimed at keeping prices high, but also through a range of other regulatory measures – all with a view to reducing consumption levels. Quite clearly, acceptance and implementation of this WHO report by Member States would necessitate a co-ordinated governmental response, and over the next decade, both in its specific alcohol proposals and in its wider health promotion activities, the WHO developed a framework which Member States could use, if they so wished, in establishing co-ordinated and comprehensive 'national alcohol policies'.[6]

When one recalls the policy approach adopted by the Intoxicating Liquor Commission 1925, the concept of a national alcohol policy appears neither original nor unrealistic in an Irish context. The question, however, is whether in the changed policy climate of the 1970s and 1980s, where alcohol consumption had become normalised, policy makers had the political will to revert to the drier policies now called for by the WHO.

In concluding this account of the emergence of the public health perspective internationally, some reference must also be made to the growing body of evidence from evaluative research that the outcomes of conventional alcoholism treatment programmes were disappointingly poor. Evaluation of the outcomes of alcoholism programmes typically involves some measure of social and emotional functioning, rather than an exclusive focus on whether or not patients remain abstinent in the post-treatment period. Alcoholism treatment, as it evolved after the Second World War, consisted largely of counselling and psychotherapy rather than pharmacotherapies, and so was not amenable to the double-blind randomised controlled trial which is the optimum research methodology used in medicine for testing the efficacy of new drug treatments.

Regardless of methodological difficulties, there was a remarkable consistency to the findings of outcome studies, and, shockingly perhaps, the main conclusion was that conventional alcoholism treatment conferred little or no therapeutic benefits on its patients. One controversial and much cited British study (Orford and Edwards, 1977), which randomly allocated newly-diagnosed alcoholics to an intensive treatment regime, including in-patient treatment for those deemed to need it and a range of drug and psychosocial therapies, or to a single out-patient session of advice-giving, at least approximated to optimum research conditions. The results of this study showed that at twelve-month follow-up there were no significant differences in outcome between the two groups; in other words, patients who were given one well-prepared session of advice, lasting for a couple of hours, did just as well as patients who had received the package of intensive and expensive therapies which was generally favoured at this time.[7]

Since the disease concept had its origins in the USA and since enthusiasm for treatment had been particularly high in that country, it is important to refer also to some American evaluative literature. One of the most highly regarded American studies of alcoholism in the post-war period was *The Natural History of Alcoholism,* the first edition of which was published in 1983. Its author, a Harvard psychiatrist, George Vaillant, was well-known for his longitudinal research into mental health and coping across the life span, but in this book his focus was exclusively on alcoholism. He describes how his interest in and commitment to alcoholism treatment grew during his clinical involvement with the *Cambridge and Somerville Program for Alcohol Rehabilitation* (CASPAR), to the point where he was satisfied that he 'was working for the most exciting alcohol program in the world'.[8] However, when he switched from a clinical to a research mode and did follow-up studies of the CASPAR patients, he found that this programme was no more successful or effective than any other. His overall conclusion was that there was no evidence that any of the conventional treatment and rehabilitation programmes added to or accelerated what he described as a commonly occurring process of natural healing or spontaneous recovery; one of his fears, in fact, was that treatment programmes might cut across and delay spontaneous recovery.

While Vaillant may have wrestled with his conscience on this issue, it should be pointed out that the overall momentum of what its critics were coming to describe as 'the alcoholism treatment industry' in the USA was in no way impeded by these negative research findings.[9] On the contrary, the concept of *recovery* was broadened to include, not just those who were dependent upon drugs or alcohol, but relatives and friends who were increasingly referred to as 'dysfunctional families', 'enablers', 'co-dependants' or 'adult children of alcoholics'.

The role of INCA during a period of attempted revisionism

In presenting an account of how the public health perspective emerged in Ireland as a challenge to the disease concept of alcoholism, an exploration of the role of the Irish National Council on Alcoholism (INCA) will be used as a convenient device for drawing together a wide range of material relating particularly to: (1) *reorienting the health services* and (2) *healthy public policy,* two of the key concepts of health promotion discussed in Chapter One.

While it might seem illogical to focus on INCA, a body which had so clearly nailed its ideological colours to the mast from its inception, there are valid reasons for so doing. The first such reason is that INCA was the only national organisation which lobbied for change in alcohol policy, and, in the absence of any specialist alcohol policy unit in the Department of Health, it had a unique opportunity to make its mark in this field. Furthermore, it was given statutory funding and formal recognition by the

Minister for Health in 1973, describing itself thereafter as a 'government-approved voluntary body'. The second reason is that INCA, from the early 1970s onwards, contained within its ranks most of those people who might be seen as the key players in this arena; these included both public-sector and private-sector psychiatrists whose views on the desirability of a continuously expanding treatment system might not necessarily coincide, as well as researchers and epidemiologists who might reasonably be expected to be familiar with the emerging public health perspective. What needs to be considered, therefore, is how INCA adapted or adjusted to the notion that it should be primarily concerned with prevention. If politicians, civil servants, the media and the general public were to be persuaded of the validity of health promotion, the persuasion was most likely to come from INCA.

The difficulty involved in this process of adjustment or transition from a curative to a preventive emphasis became apparent in 1973, at the very moment when INCA had all the appearance of being on the crest of a wave. In October 1971, INCA had held a conference in Dun Laoghaire which attracted the interest of the then Tánaiste and Minister for Health, Erskine Childers. Unlike Seán Flanagan, his predecessor, Erskine Childers was wholeheartedly and unequivocally committed to the disease concept and believed that the time was ripe for a serious policy initiative in this area. He also thought that such an initiative should be co-ordinated by INCA, and one of his officials wrote as follows to the Chairman of INCA, Mr Justice Cearbhall Ó Dálaigh:

> The Tánaiste is anxious that the interest and enthusiasm created by the recent Conference should not be allowed to disappear and he wishes to know, therefore, what are the views of INCA as to what our next steps should be. He visualises that INCA should consult with others engaged in this field who should be given an opportunity of submitting such evidence as they may see fit.
>
> We have no definite guidelines to lay down as to how you should tackle this task but what we have in mind is that you should examine the problem, in the light of the knowledge gleaned from the Conference, and consider in broad outline what practical action you would recommend for the immediate future.[10]

In response to this request INCA spent the whole of 1972 in a process of consultation and discussion, following which a lengthy report was submitted to the Minister for Health in January 1973. In setting out in summary form its recommendations for 'publicity and propaganda', the report put explicit emphasis on the value of 'stressing the disease concept and thereby removing the stigma of alcoholism, in order to encourage the acceptance of treatment at an early stage'.[11] However, the copy of the report subsequently available at INCA headquarters contained the following footnote:

> There is a minority viewpoint that over-emphasis on the disease concept has grave disadvantages in that it concentrates too much on individual susceptibility and fails to recognise that quantity, frequency and the use that alcohol is put to by the individual are of greater importance. Moreover, by stressing the disease concept there is the implication that these factors are NOT important. (This footnote was added in November 1973 subsequent to the submission of the Report to the Minister for Health).[12]

A similar footnote records the suggestion that all alcohol beverage containers should carry a Government warning to the effect that 'This beverage contains alcohol and is therefore liable to produce dependence';[13] this footnote was also omitted from the Minister's copy, as was another suggestion that wives of alcoholics should be given free legal aid if they wished to separate from husbands whose drinking disrupted family life and caused emotional damage to children.[14]

These footnotes, omitted from the copy given to the Minister, clearly suggest that within INCA an alternative perspective was emerging at this time. The decision to conceal from the Minister the existence of ideological disagreement of such a fundamental kind is completely understandable in the light of INCA's obvious determination to use this opportunity to achieve more formal recognition and financial support from the Minister. The Minister's enthusiasm for INCA was almost certainly based on the apparent consensus attaching to the disease concept, and might not have survived a report which dealt openly with ideological conflict and which highlighted the associated policy dilemmas. However prudent it may have been for INCA to present a united front at this particular juncture, it still left the organisation with the difficult task of deciding where it stood in relation to the two polarised paradigms: the disease concept and the public health perspective. Would INCA, as the expert advisory body on these matters, continue to urge the Minister for Health to develop curative services or would it lobby for a multisectoral alcohol control system in accordance with the public health perspective?

Reorienting the health services

The task of 'reorienting health services' was one of the five principal tasks of health promotion identified in the Ottawa Charter. Whether INCA had the capacity to act as an effective advocate of this process of reorientation was always in doubt because of the dominant position of doctors, and of psychiatrists in particular, in its membership. It would be naïve to expect doctors, whose authority and financial security were overwhelmingly based upon curative service provision, to transform themselves overnight into lobbyists for a preventive system in which the validity and effectiveness of curative services were seriously questioned.

However, the doctors within INCA did not function as a homogeneous group articulating a common or 'party' line. One source of disagreement which manifested itself periodically was the tension between public and private medicine. Alcoholism admissions to the Irish psychiatric system had risen steadily since the mid-1960s to a point in the late-1970s where they accounted for a quarter of all admissions. A health policy paper which was published by the National Economic and Social Council (NESC) in 1983 commented critically on this trend, pointing out that whereas alcoholism had accounted for 25 per cent of all psychiatric admissions in Ireland during 1979, it had accounted for less than 7 per cent of English admissions for the same year.[15] However, if one breaks down the Irish mental health admission statistics by type of hospital (and, broadly speaking, there are three types of in-patient system – *health board hospitals, general hospital psychiatric units* and *private psychiatric hospitals*), it becomes clear that alcoholism admissions were a great deal more common in private psychiatric hospitals than in either of the other two systems. For instance in 1979, the year selected by NESC for comparative purposes, alcoholism admissions accounted for 40 per cent of private hospital admissions, but only 23 per cent of health board admissions.[16]

Understandably, psychiatrists from the private hospitals were unlikely to undermine what was an important therapeutic and commercial function of these institutions by using INCA to lobby for a radical reorientation of the health services, away from treatment towards prevention. There were, however, some public sector psychiatrists in INCA who did not subscribe fully to the disease concept or to its associated enthusiasm for treatment. The opinions which were consigned to footnotes in INCA's report of 1973 and deemed unsuitable for the eyes of the Minister for Health were those of Dr R.D. Stevenson, a consultant psychiatrist with the Eastern Health Board and clinical director of St Dymphna's Hospital, the largest health board alcoholism treatment unit in the country. Dr Stevenson had become a member of INCA within a few years of its establishment but soon became disaffected with the disease concept, arguing that it depicted alcohol in an excessively benign light, excused irresponsible drinking and made unrealistic claims for the efficacy of alcoholism treatment.[17]

Another fault line within INCA lay in the differing perspectives between those doctors who were solely or principally clinicians and those who were committed to research. In this latter category, the two members of INCA who were most consistently and explicitly to champion the public health perspective and to question the wisdom of putting resources into specialist treatment services were Dr Geoffrey Dean, Director of the Medico-Social Research Board, and Dr Dermot Walsh who was in charge of mental health epidemiology in the same institute.[18]

Because of his many publications, it is relatively easy to trace Dermot Walsh's increasing scepticism with and eventual repudiation of the disease concept. At the INCA Conference which was held in Dun Laoghaire in 1971, Professor Norman Moore, who was Medical Director of St Patrick's Hospital and a founder member of INCA, summarised and drew recommendations from the overall proceedings. Norman Moore's perspective is best exemplified in his statement that: 'The nature of the physical change [involved in alcoholism] is unknown, but its solution, I believe, lies with the laboratory scientists. One day I think they will give us the answer.' In a further comment referring to the lack of research in this country, Moore went on to say that: 'Dr Dermot Walsh's research into the field of addiction problems in Ireland has been a splendid exception to the general criticism concerning the lack of research'.[19] Approbation from this source was understandable at this time because Dermot Walsh still subscribed to the disease concept, albeit with some scepticism. In a 1972 paper, for instance, Walsh was still broadly positive about the increased numbers of patients being admitted to hospital for alcoholism; he wrote:

> In Local Authority hospitals the first admission increase from 1965 to 1969 was from 258 first admissions to 560 first admissions, an increase of 117 per cent; whereas for private hospitals the increase was from 441 first admissions to 621, an increase of 41 per cent. This confirms that a greater number of working class people are accepting treatment in Local Authority hospitals and that it is this increase in working class admissions which accounts for the greater part of the 69 per cent increase observed from 1965 to 1969. If this hypothesis is true it represents a very rapid and heartening change for the good in the changed community attitude towards alcoholism and the willingness of persons to seek treatment for the condition. Whether treatments will prove effective is something which we cannot evaluate at the moment ...

Over the next few years, however, through his work in the Medico-Social Research Board and his international consultancy and research, Dermot Walsh was increasingly drawn into the network of those who advocated the public health perspective, coming in the process to reject unequivocally the disease concept.

In 1976, for instance, the European Regional Office of the WHO, in conjunction with the Addiction Research Foundation of Toronto, initiated an international study of alcohol problems and the role of the state in controlling or preventing such problems. This study, known as the International Study of Alcohol Control Experiences (ISACE), involved seven 'states': Poland, Finland, Switzerland, Holland, Ireland, Ontario and California. Dermot Walsh, together with the economist Dr Brendan Walsh, represented Ireland on this project; his participation in ISACE was, however, on behalf of the Medico-Social Research Board rather than INCA, and in this role he became explicitly critical of INCA and its commitment to the disease concept. This detailed, critical perspective is captured, for example, in one of the ISACE publications in which Dermot and Brendan Walsh commented on how drinking problems were then perceived in Ireland:

> At the same time, there is an increasing tendency, due to the efforts of various bodies such as the Irish National Council on Alcoholism, Alcoholics Anonymous, and the medical profession, to regard alcoholism as a 'disease'. This conceptualisation leads to a different type of permissiveness, in that it implies an inability to control drinking rather than an unwillingness to do so. At the same time, many wives as well as husbands see in this disease concept of alcoholism the legitimisation of a man's heavy drinking and the condoning of behaviour that otherwise would be condemned.[20]

It is clear, therefore, that INCA was not in a position to advise the Minister for Health unequivocally on this issue of alcoholism treatment; its internal ideological split on this matter simply made this an impossibility. What appears to have happened from the mid-1970s is that an uneasy truce prevailed within INCA on the subject of alcoholism treatment: those who favoured the curative approach were less vociferous than they might have been, while those who were critical also restrained themselves, so that the agency avoided overt conflict and survived. While this tactic of peaceful coexistence guaranteed INCA's survival, it also (as will be shown later in this section) greatly hindered its ability to act as an effective lobbyist for the remainder of its organisational life.

An additional complication was the importation into Ireland of a new American treatment model, commonly referred to as the *Minnesota Model.* This particular variant of the disease concept had evolved, as its name suggests, in the State of Minnesota, where from the 1950s onwards it was particularly espoused by organisations such as the Hazelden Foundation and the Johnson Institute.[21] It represented a professionalisation of the therapeutic philosophy and methods of AA, but differed fundamentally from AA in its advocacy of confrontation as a therapeutic tool and also in its espousal of highly structured in-patient programmes with lengthy aftercare. To those who believed that treatment should be de-emphasised in Irish health policy, the Minnesota Model represented a most untimely evangelical argument for the retention and expansion of curative services.

If the Roman Catholic Church in Ireland had been slow to warm to the disease concept, it more than compensated for this delay by the alacrity it displayed in promoting the Minnesota Model. Almost without exception, it was priests and nuns who advanced the cause of the Minnesota Model and, by comparison with the vacillation of INCA, their work in this regard was an object lesson in effective lobbying. Why the Minnesota Model should have been so attractive to Irish religious at this time is not absolutely clear. This was a time when members of religious orders became interested in doing pastoral work outside what had been their mainstream activities in the educational and healthcare systems, and addiction treatment – particularly when it made such explicit use of spiritual themes as was the case with the Minnesota Model – appears to have been seen as a new and highly appropriate form of pastoral care. In any event, the first Irish treatment programme to be set up on these lines was at the Stanhope Social Service Centre in the north inner-city of Dublin; this was a structured out-patient programme which was created in 1976 by Sr Marie Joseph O'Reilly of the Irish Sisters of Charity, modelled on the programme she had trained in at St Mary's Hospital in Minneapolis and run with financial support from the Eastern Health Board.

However, a much greater impact on the treatment scene in Ireland was made by the opening in early 1978 of the Rutland Centre, an in-patient unit which was set up in a disused convent in Clondalkin, Dublin, with accommodation for twenty-four clients. The Rutland Centre offered an intensive and highly-structured treatment programme, with an average in-patient stay of six weeks, followed by a two-year aftercare period. This centre was set up by Fr Raphael Short, a priest of the Passionist Order, who had qualified in clinical psychology and subsequently spent some time in the USA, training in the use of the Minnesota Model. In 1977, Fr Short approached the Minister for Health, Charles Haughey, with a request for financial support for his proposed treatment centre. The submission to the Minister was couched in the usual terms of the Minnesota Model, describing the addicted person as 'out of touch with reality' and, through its emphasis on the 'drug-free' nature of the proposed treatment methods, implicitly criticising the existing medical approach to addiction treatment in Ireland. Fr Short's proposal was unambiguously clear and optimistic:

> Drawing on the experience and success of similar centres in the United States, particularly in the State of Minnesota and assisted by their personnel, this centre hopes to offer an alternative form of alcoholism treatment which is drug free and based on the principles of crisis intervention and Reality Therapy. Where the model operates in the United States, a recovery rate of 60-70 per cent is claimed, based on a criterion of three years sobriety from the date of discharge.[22]

If the Department of Health had a specialist policy unit dealing with alcohol issues, or if it had received clear policy advice from INCA questioning the claimed 'success rates' or discouraging it from financing this new development, the Minister might have rejected Fr Short's submission. What happened, however, was that the Minister agreed to provide £23,000 from the Hospital Trust Fund towards the capital costs of the new centre and £70,000 per annum from the health budget for staff salaries. The Rutland Centre was regarded as a pilot project which would be monitored for two years, following which the Department of Health and the Eastern Health Board would reconsider financial support for this venture.

The Eastern Health Board debated the establishment of the Rutland Centre at its meeting of 12 January 1978, although the reality of the situation was that Mr Haughey's commitment to this project effectively presented the Board with a *fait accompli*. Enthusiasm for the Rutland Centre was muted, to say the least, and from the minutes of this meeting (and from general recall of this period) it is possible to discern a sense of shock that somebody who was not a medical doctor should seek and be granted considerable health funding for an alcoholism treatment centre. Statistics provided for this meeting of the Eastern Health Board suggested that the Board's own specialist alcoholism unit, St Dymphna's, was both dealing with a much larger number of patients than the Rutland Centre could ever aspire to cater for *and* providing a more comprehensive service (including detoxification and other medical care). The annual cost of the St Dymphna's service was approximately £100,000, while the projected annual cost of the Rutland Centre was £120,000. In the circumstances, there was something almost pathetically revealing about the comment in the minutes of this meeting to the effect that: 'A request by Dr Stevenson [Clinical Director of St Dymphna's] for additional support staff is being examined'.[23] What this suggested was that the Eastern Health Board was experiencing difficulties in providing its own long-established alcoholism unit with the level of resources it was thought to require, while at the same time acting, on Ministerial orders, as a conduit for the payment of substantial funding to a new voluntary agency, concerning which it had many reservations.

A final example of the misgivings of the conventional healthcare system and the medical profession towards these interlopers, into what had been an exclusively medical domain, may be found in the contribution to this meeting of Professor Stephen Doyle, a physician at St Lawrence's Hospital and a member at this time of the Eastern Health Board. Professor Doyle expressed great reservations about the Rutland Centre on the grounds that it proposed to detoxify alcoholics without having the services of a full-time doctor; he pointed out that *delirium tremens* had a mortality rate of ten per cent and that 'to treat it in Clondalkin made a big "medical hole" in the proposals'.[24] This objection was quickly made to appear spurious when Fr Short wrote to each member of the Board pointing out that it had never been intended to detoxify patients in the Rutland Centre, which was after all a drug-free facility, but that patients would be admitted only after they had been detoxified elsewhere under medical supervision.[25]

In any event, the Rutland Centre was opened for business in early 1978 and its official opening was performed by Mr Haughey on 17 May of that year. It proved to be merely the first in a line of Minnesota-style residential units which would open in Ireland over the next twenty years, all of which would contribute to the further popularisation of the disease concept, at a time when the WHO and other health-care authorities were calling for a transfer of resources and energies to health promotion. One of the innovations associated with this new American-style treatment system, which was commented upon by the Minister for Health in his address at the opening of the Rutland Centre, was the emergence of a new treatment professional, the *alcoholism counsellor.* In the USA these counsellors were mainly alcoholics who were in 'recovery', but in Ireland the picture was rather more mixed, with nurses, social workers and other professionals displaying an enthusiasm for this new title. Obviously, the emergence of this new professional group – almost exclusively committed to the curative perspective and to 'recovery' – militated further against the growth of a health promotional or preventive perspective on alcohol in Ireland.

Another consequence of the advent of the Minnesota Model was the broadening of the client population to include spouses, children and other family members and friends of alcoholics, all of whom were drawn into the therapeutic net on the basis that alcoholism was a 'family disease' or that those close to the alcoholic could frequently be classified as 'enablers' or 'co-dependants'. Perhaps the most extreme example of this trend was the growing popularity of the label of ACOA (Adult Child of an Alcoholic); this reflected the belief that adults who had grown up in the care of an alcoholic parent were frequently, if not invariably, subject to life-long emotional and personality difficulties and so in need of specific and on-going treatment or support.

There is no evidence that either in relation to the funding of the Rutland Centre or to the wider topic of the Minnesota Model the Department of Health ever consulted INCA. This new American approach to alcoholism treatment did not, on the face of it, have the support of either of the two dissenting factions within INCA: those opposed to the disease concept were unlikely to be enthusiastic about what was, essentially, a new and evangelical version of this concept, while those still committed to a curative perspective were dubious about a model which was not under the control of the medical profession and which threatened to poach customers away from the private hospital sector. INCA made no policy pronouncements on this development, almost certainly because of its own unresolved internal conflicts. However, Fr Short and subsequent advocates of the Minnesota Model displayed an approach to lobbying which would be referred to in Irish as *an modh díreach:* they made direct, unapologetic approaches to those in a position to fund their services, arguing for the self-evident value of this model and, as often as not, they succeeded. Had INCA been functioning as a coherent body, capable of dispassionate policy analysis and advice, it might have pointed out to the Minister for Health that claims for the efficacy of the Minnesota Model were exaggerated and were certainly not based upon conventional scientific research; it might also have drawn the Minister's attention to the evolving public health perspective and the *volte face* of the WHO on this topic. Even had it done so, however, there is no reason to believe that INCA would have dissuaded the Minister for Health from his support for what appeared to be a popular development in the area of treatment services.

The disagreement and lack of common purpose which characterised INCA became particularly clear in the spring of 1985, when two policy developments in the alcoholism treatment area were announced (coincidentally, it appears) at about the same time. The first of these was the publication of *The Psychiatric Services: Planning for the Future,* the final report of a study group appointed by the Minister for Health in 1981 to draw up guidelines for the development of the country's mental health services. *Planning for the Future* (as this report is commonly described) was made public in March 1985 and was subsequently accepted as the official policy blueprint for public psychiatric services in Ireland for the foreseeable future. In relation to alcohol, *Planning for the Future* advocated a health promotional or public health perspective which will be discussed in the next section of this chapter. In relation to alcoholism treatment, however, the report unequivocally denounced the prevalence of psychiatric in-patient treatment as being excessively high, given the results of evaluative research which indicated that brief community-based interventions were as effective as lengthy in-patient treatment. The alternative to in-patient treatment which *Planning for the Future* proposed was the establishment of community alcohol services within the sectorised mental health system. The concept of sectorisation refers to the administrative rearrangement of public mental health services, involving the delivery of services to designated geographic catchment areas, or sectors, by mental health teams headed by consultant psychiatrists. While it was conceded that specialist alcoholism counselling should be retained, it was recommended that counsellors should be integrated as far as possible into the sector teams.[26]

The second policy development in this area was the decision by the Voluntary Health Insurance (VHI) organisation to limit its insurance cover of in-patient treatment for alcoholism and drug dependence. In March 1985, as part of its annual renewal procedures, VHI began to inform subscribers that henceforth in-patient cover of alcoholism treatment would be limited to two admissions, not exceeding 42 days each and with at least 180 days between them. In addition to this limitation, VHI also announced that all hospital cover was to be reduced to a maximum of 180 days *per annum* and that maternity cover was to be reduced, for routine deliveries, from seven to five days. Although there was considerable media coverage and public discussion of all these changes in the VHI scheme, by far the greatest controversy arose in relation to the alcoholism treatment changes.

Claims for in-patient alcoholism treatment at this time were consistently less than one per cent of all claims received annually by the VHI, but their significance lay in the length of stay involved and also in the high rate of readmission. Average length of stay in general hospitals (for VHI claims) in 1985 was 8 days; for psychiatric admissions (excluding alcoholism) average length of stay for this year was 48 days, and for alcoholism admissions it was 30 days.[27] The VHI decision to reduce its cover of alcoholism treatment not only corresponded to the policy advocated in *Planning for the Future,* but also brought the organisation closer to the norm which was evolving within American health insurance companies, which by this time was tending to provide cover for just a single in-patient rehabilitation programme of 28 days duration.

INCA made no public pronouncements about either of these two policy developments. Dermot Walsh had been a member of the study group which produced *Planning for the Future;* his epidemiological data were a central feature of this report and his overall determination to reduce rates of hospitalisation and lengths of stay was evident throughout the report. The private-sector psychiatrists within INCA might be indifferent to the proposed changes in the treatment of alcoholism in public hospitals, but they were certainly not indifferent to the proposed changes in VHI's financing of alcoholism treatment in their own sphere.

A 'straw poll' reported by the *Irish Medical Times* in early April 1985 showed that psychiatrists in private hospitals were unanimous in their condemnation of this VHI change, while their colleagues in the public health sector were ambivalent, with some giving clear approval to these limitations on in-patient cover. The flavour of the debate at this time may be gleaned from the press coverage of a public lecture at St Patrick's Hospital:

> Dr John Cooney, Associate Medical Director of St Patrick's Hospital, said in a
> lecture on 'The Problem Drinker' that the VHI's measures were quite arbitrary

and could not be justified, given the natural history of alcoholism and the necessity for properly organised treatment programming designed to achieve recovery rather than mere sobriety.

The VHI organisation would appear to be unaware of the major advances in treatment of latter years in this country, with consequent restoration to health and happiness of so many alcoholics and their families ...

It was also highly disquieting to contemplate the prospect of the alcoholic being forced to go underground and conceal his or her problem, after all these years of painstaking and often frustrating endeavour to remove the stigma of alcoholism.[28]

On the other hand, in a rare and mischievous public statement of the view that private psychiatric hospitals were part of the problem rather than part of the solution, Sr Marie Joseph, who had founded the Stanhope Street Alcoholism Centre and who subscribed to the Minnesota Model, wrote:

During my more than 20 years of work with alcoholics I have found the greatest obstacle to their recovery to be the people who take responsibility for them and provide for their comforts. No better place to do both than in the private hospital.

If alcoholics are kept secure and comfortable they won't stop drinking no matter how much they want to. They can't. The best help that can be given is to expose them to the full consequences of their drinking.

To the VHI I would say: 'You have done a good day's work! Stick to it!'[29]

It is important to note, however, that publicly aired disagreements of this kind were merely about the relative merits of one form of alcoholism treatment as opposed to another, rather than about whether treatment as a whole should play a subsidiary role to health promotion – which is what *Planning for the Future* had advocated.

During this period of public debate about the VHI changes, INCA once again played no direct role and issued no public statement on this topic. A few months prior to this, one of the Executive Directors of INCA, Mr Shane Gray, had told a Council meeting that 'the absence of a clear policy in some areas, and lack of consensus among Council members on particular issues, made it difficult sometimes to respond satisfactorily to media enquiries'.[30] Clearly, the issue of VHI changes with regard to alcoholism treatment was a case in point, but in the absence of Dermot Walsh – who had indicated that he was 'not in full agreement'[31] with a draft response to VHI which had been circulated to members – a relatively mild letter of protest was sent to VHI on the matter.

There were in fact decreases in the numbers of alcoholics being hospitalised following the acceptance and implementation of *Planning for the Future*. These decreases consisted of reductions both in absolute numbers and in alcohol admissions expressed as a proportion of all mental health admissions, but they were relatively modest, slow to materialise, and could not be taken as evidence of any major 'reorientation of the health services' in this sphere. It must be concluded, therefore, that during the period 1973-1988 INCA did not consistently and successfully advocate or lobby for a reorientation of health services – where this phrase refers to a downplaying of the importance of curative services relative to prevention or health promotion. While it included in its membership some professionals, such as Dermot Walsh and Geoffrey Dean, who were keen advocates of the emerging public health perspective, INCA also contained many members who were totally committed to traditional alcoholism treatment: its ambivalence on the issue was also reflected in the fact that, during the revitalisation of the treatment system which followed the advent of the Minnesota Model, it sought and received from the Department of Health what amounted to a monopoly on the training and accreditation of alcoholism counsellors.

Building healthy public policy

The concept of 'building healthy public policy' is another of the concepts identified in the Ottawa Charter as being central to the general health promotion project. In the context of alcohol and its associated problems, healthy public policy essentially refers to the drafting and implementation of comprehensive national alcohol policies, as advocated by public health activists generally and by the WHO specifically. The fundamental belief which underlies this perspective is that alcohol, although a legal and culturally acceptable drug, is toxic, addictive and implicated in a wide range of social and behavioural problems; consequently, it is argued, the most rational and effective way to lower the incidence and prevalence of alcohol-related problems is to reduce consumption. Healthy public policy is intended to involve the co-ordinated activities of all sectors of government in achieving this ambition, and not just the health sector activity. Thus, for example, the education sector might be expected to inform the public (and young people in particular) of the link between individual consumption levels and risk; the law enforcement sector might be expected to enforce all aspects of a tough licensing system which curtailed access to alcohol; and finance and revenue sectors might be expected to use fiscal measures to reduce or limit consumption rather than as a tool to maximise revenue for the Exchequer or to create jobs. A summary of this healthy public policy approach to the prevention of alcohol-related problems was contained in Chapter 13 of *Planning for the Future,* along with the view that INCA as 'the primary advisory body in the field of alcohol-related problems in this country'[32] should be involved in the formulation of a national alcohol policy.

When one considers how difficult INCA found it to handle the specific issue of treatment policy, there is no reason to expect that it would perform more coherently or effectively in the general alcohol policy area. The difficulties facing INCA in advocating healthy public policy stemmed both from its own internal organisational difficulties and from the external policy climate. The internal issues, of course, refer to the lack of ideological consensus which characterised the organisation from 1973 onwards: it is reasonable to assume that the main support for healthy public policy came from those few Council members with research interests, while members who were primarily committed to clinical services may have been less interested in preventive activity on the grand scale envisaged here. The external factors consist principally of the opposition to alcohol control policies which could be anticipated from the general public, from the drinks industry and from other sectors of government.

It was argued at the conclusion of Chapter Two that the great strength of the disease concept lay in its universal appeal rather than in any inherent scientific validity: it was popular with the public because it suggested that only those who were 'alcoholic' needed to exercise caution in their drinking habits; popular with the drinks industry for the same reason; and popular with clinicians because it encouraged the growth of a vibrant treatment industry. In its attempt to sell the public health perspective and the necessity for healthy public policy in the alcohol sphere, INCA may have had access to supporting scientific data of a reputable kind, but it is difficult to conceive of a more unpopular policy line than that which flowed from this research. The message to the public was that all drinkers – and not just heavy drinkers or dependent drinkers – should be circumspect in their drinking habits; indeed some proponents of the public health perspective argued that all drinkers, regardless of their consumption levels, should reduce their consumption by one-third. Worse still, the concept of healthy public policy did not rely solely, or even primarily, on techniques of persuasion to alter drinking habits, but argued for control policies (such as price increases, curtailment of access to retail outlets and bans on alcohol advertising and promotion) which had an undeniably paternalistic air to them. In ideological terms, the concept of co-ordinated national alcohol policies was generally described by representatives of the international drinks trade as a form of neo-prohibitionism or 'health fascism', although high-minded, libertarian rhetoric of this kind could never really conceal their underlying fear for their profit margins. Finally, it would be unrealistic to expect sectors of government which were primarily concerned with the revenue-generating or job-creation aspects of the drinks industry to have any great welcome for healthy public policy in this sphere.

To what extent then did INCA succeed in reconciling its own internal ideological differences in relation to healthy public policy, and what strategy did it use in seeking to persuade legislators and central government officials of the validity of this policy? The clearest evidence that INCA did somehow revise its thinking and shift from its original neutrality on the subject of alcohol is to be found in two policy documents which were prepared in 1979 and 1980; the 1979 document was a submission to the Minister for Health, while the 1980 document was a submission to the Minister for Justice. The submission to the Minister for Health was a short document which summarised the data and conclusions from the influential *Alcohol Control Policies in Public Health Perspective*. The message to the Minister for Health was summarised succinctly as follows: 'Changes in the overall consumption of alcoholic beverages have a bearing on the health of the people in any society. Alcohol control measures can be used to limit consumption; thus control of alcohol becomes a public health issue'.[33] The submission to the Minister for Justice was somewhat lengthier and drew heavily on research from the Medico-Social Research Board; it concentrated on the prospects of using licensing legislation and road traffic legislation to reduce dangerous alcohol consumption and its conclusion was:

> Since the prevalence of alcoholism and other alcohol-related problems increases with the growth of consumption of alcohol at national level, control of availability is an essential feature of preventive measures.
> Control can be exercised by limiting access to alcohol itself – particularly to young people – and by revising and enforcing legislation, as suggested in this paper.[34]

Both of these documents obviously represented an ideological shift for INCA from its earlier preoccupation with alcoholism and its treatment; they were nonetheless moderate statements of the public health perspective, lacking stridency or emotionalism, and their emphasis on young people's drinking – a topic on which there tends to be almost universal albeit bland consensus – helped to diminish any sense of neo-prohibitionism which might otherwise be attributed to them. Regardless of the content of these two documents, however, the strategy adopted by INCA in lobbying for political acceptance of this approach is equally in need of scrutiny. In fact, the decision taken by INCA was to send these documents to the two Ministers and to follow this up with direct meetings with the Ministers or, more hopefully, a series of meetings in which the research basis for and the practical value of the public health perspective could be spelt out. The view within INCA was that the Council was a reputable and respected body (it had, incidentally, strong connections with both the Fianna Fáil and Fine Gael parties) which could use its status to lobby discreetly for policy change in this area. Neither of the two submissions was published and no public pronouncement of any kind was made on this change of policy within INCA; indeed to members of the public who gave any thought to this subject it must have appeared as though the organisation still adhered to the disease concept, which had been advocated so cogently and publicly by its first Director.

The decision to rely on direct lobbying at a high level, rather than to publicise these issues through the media, appears to have failed completely, since successive ministers simply did not meet INCA representatives or treat them with the gravity and deference which they seemed to regard as their due. The strategy was criticised retrospectively by Dr R.D. Stevenson, who told this writer repeatedly that he regarded it as a mistake not to have lobbied publicly and actively on this front, and in 1986 he wrote: 'We all give an impression of deep concern for the public welfare. But we have had zero influence on the course of events because we have never rocked the boat. We have always gone through normal channels'.[35] In theoretical terms, the INCA strategy corresponds closely to the *organisational networks* model, one of the three models of policy co-ordination described by Harrison and Tether, which was summarised in Chapter One. It was not inevitably a losing strategy: if INCA had the commitment and the political skills to use its contacts with politicians, senior civil servants, the churches, the media and others it might well have succeeded in achieving some elements at least of a public health policy. It is instructive to remember how advocates of the Minnesota Model had made direct and usually profitable contact with politicians. By contrast, INCA attempts to 'network' with Ministers, senior civil servants and other influential players in this arena appear to have been excessively genteel and inept, and to have made virtually no progress.

Reading through INCA papers from the period 1979 to 1988, one cannot escape the conclusion that, in large measure, its failure to act as an effective advocate of the public health perspective stemmed from the fact that the organisation itself was half-hearted and ambivalent on this issue. It would be wrong to see the two submissions which have been discussed as representing a consensus within the Council, or as representing an agenda which was being actively and consistently pursued. Instead, the reality was that INCA throughout this period remained in a state of ideological confusion and ambiguity, and was also in an increasingly moribund state organisationally with meetings being held infrequently and little business being conducted. The minutes of the Council meeting for 24 September, 1984, for example, included a summary of a discussion concerning the relationship between INCA and the Health Education

Bureau; it is clear from this excerpt just how ambiguous INCA was in its pursuit of the public health perspective at this time:

> Mrs O'Hagan suggested that the Council has always been concerned with 'alcoholism' while the Bureau have [sic] also been concerned with 'alcohol'.
> Dr Dean suggested that INCA had always emphasised the disease concept of alcoholism – a concept which was particularly acceptable to the drinks industry ... He believed the Council should state clearly that its objective was to reduce consumption.[36]

Despite engaging in periodic reviews and attempts to regain a clear focus as to its *raison d'être,* INCA failed to renew itself or to regain the consensus which had characterised its early years. It ultimately appeared to fall between two stools in the sense that it never fully committed itself to the public health perspective, although it also lost its close contacts with AA and with those who still subscribed to the disease concept. An attempt in 1984 by one of its Directors, Mrs Mary O'Hagan, to establish a formal link with the Hazelden Foundation of Minnesota became the occasion of a rather embarrassing critique of INCA. Hazelden is the largest and best-known of the foundations which promotes the Minnesota Model, and Mrs O'Hagan had hoped that it would be interested in setting up a formal collaboration with INCA which would involve Hazelden in the training of Irish alcoholism counsellors, while INCA would also act as a distribution agent for Hazelden educational and training materials. A report from Mrs O'Hagan to INCA outlined the stringent criteria laid down by Hazelden's representative, Mr Gordon Grimm, at a meeting which took place in June, 1984. In summary, Hazelden was reluctant to become involved with any organisation which was not 'highly dynamic' and obviously influential in its own community; it also favoured the involvement of 'recovering alcoholics' at a senior level. 'He [Mr Grimm] asked how often the Council and Executive Committee met, and remarked that the fact that the Council had not met since the last AGM would not indicate particular commitment as far as Hazelden was concerned'.[37] Not surprisingly, nothing came of this venture.

One of the few occasions on which INCA appears to have become engaged in direct and explicit lobbying for the introduction of alcohol control policies occurred in 1984 when there was a review of the licensing laws by the Joint Committee on Legislation. Following a written submission to the Joint Committee, INCA was invited to make an oral submission and did so through its two Directors, Mrs Mary O'Hagan and Mr Shane Gray. The responses of the Dáil Deputies and Senators suggest that they were unfamiliar with this new policy line being advocated by the INCA representatives, and that they were both surprised and unhappy at the importance which was now being attached to control systems. Deputy Desmond O'Malley quoted from the statistics, supplied by INCA, which compared alcohol consumption rates internationally, and asked the two INCA representatives and a representative from the Pioneer Total Abstinence Association what all the fuss was about:

> We all express great concern about the level of it, the dangers and the difficulties. We consider it very bad here. I would have thought it was bad and I would have thought it was getting worse. Look at it, we are almost the most liquor free country in Europe. We are .9 of a litre above the very bottom in terms of absolute alcohol and our decrease since 1980 in the consumption of alcohol is greater than all other countries except one. We started near the bottom and we are even nearer to the bottom now. I must confess those figures are rather heartening but they tend to conflict with the general picture that is painted. How would your two organisations reconcile these figures with the general picture and the certain degree of pessimism that there is in regard to alcoholic consumption?[38]

Shane Gray responded to this by pointing out how *per capita* consumption rates lead to crude comparisons because of differing age structures and abstinence rates, but the overall tone of the members' responses was sceptical and dismissive. This is best summed up in the remarks of Senator Shane Ross, who with Deputy Alan Shatter, was most critical of the demand for coercive, paternalistic alcohol policies:

> There is a certain emphasis on restriction in the document which the INCA produced and to a certain extent it treats people as children in saying 'This is good for you; this is bad for you!' There is an emphasis on penalties. I would endorse what Deputy Shatter said: where the emphasis should come is on education and not on restrictions. Whatever restrictions you introduce will be widely abused.[39]

There is a certain irony in this response to INCA, since it so closely resembles the policy line which INCA itself had advocated for the first few years of its existence, namely, that alcohol as a substance cannot be villified; that aggregate consumption levels are unimportant, and that education is a much more appropriate preventive tool than coercion. Ostensibly, INCA had been using its top-level contacts and its general reputation to lobby for the public health perspective for at least five years before the Joint Committee on Legislation addressed itself to the licensing legislation; the response of the politicians on this occasion suggested, however, that they had not previously heard of this approach and, furthermore, that it was unwelcome.

In 1981 a formal umbrella organisation known as the Drinks Industry

Group (DIG), representing both manufacturers and retailers, was established with a view to unifying and strengthening the voice of the industry. While the public health perspective and its proponents could scarcely take credit for it, the fact was (as Desmond O'Malley had noted) that *per capita* alcohol consumption levels – which had doubled between 1960 and 1980 – began to drop in 1980. The DIG was determined to combat the negative image of alcohol now being portrayed by public health advocates, and to oppose the notion that the state should use fiscal or other control measures to reduce consumption levels. A number of research reports and consultancy documents were prepared for the DIG, mainly by Professor John O'Hagan of the Department of Economics at Trinity College, Dublin, to further the industry's cause.[40] These reports, some of which were made public and used for advertising and promotional purposes, generally sought to undermine the public health perspective by illustrating the economic significance of the drinks industry and challenging what was seen to be an already excessive burden of taxation on alcoholic beverages. Philosophically, as one would expect from an economist, the notion of using fiscal policy to limit consumer behaviour was regarded as an unwarranted interference with consumer sovereignty. Practically, it was contended that alcohol was 'price inelastic', which means that demand is relatively insensitive to price and that demand for the commodity would not reduce automatically following a price increase; on this basis, it was argued that price increases might merely result in consumers spending more money on alcohol rather than consuming less, which in turn might add to the social costs of drinking rather than reduce them.

It was conceded that there are 'negative externalities', or costs which society as a whole must bear as a consequence of allowing individuals relative freedom to consume alcohol, but economists have generally argued that these costs to the Exchequer are more than covered by the high taxes levied on Irish drinkers.

The experience of INCA in attempting to persuade the Ministers for Justice and Health to adopt alcohol policies of a somewhat 'drier' nature is not, of course, unique in the international scene. A special 1993 issue of the journal *Addiction* dealt exclusively with the interaction between alcohol researchers and policy makers and, through a series of case studies from Europe, North America and Australia, showed how researchers had achieved, at best, limited success in this venture. An interesting and provocative paper by Secker, an Australian public sector manager who had worked for two and a half years as Director of Liquor Licensing in Western Australia, set out to explore why, 'although reasonably conclusive research exists on several topics in the liquor availability field, research has had a very limited direct impact on policy formulation'.[41] Secker suggests that generally alcohol researchers do not understand the policy formulation process or the motives and thinking of the main actors who are involved in this process. His views on Government ministers and their approach to alcohol policy formulation are presented here (Table 5) in a summarised version which, while undoubtedly patronising and stereotypical, go some way to explaining the relative success of those who lobbied for an expanded treatment sector and the almost total failure of those who lobbied for healthy public policy.

Table 5: Assumptions about government ministers which may safely be made by alcohol researchers

- They drink liquor (often heavily) and any suggestion in research that liquor consumption should be reduced might be viewed as implied criticism of their habits.
- They want good news and no bad news.
- They are pragmatic seekers of the best balance of forces playing on them at that time.
- They are short-term thinkers and prefer proposals that have clear, short-term benefits.
- They cannot understand research or statistical methodology, and are often not convinced by conclusions even if they do understand them.
- They are poor finishers – once a decision is made and the pressure is off, they lose interest in the decision and move on to the next topic.

Source: Adapted from Secker (1993)

Politicians who provide money for new alcoholism treatment services, whether or not there is research evidence as to the efficacy of such services, are gratified by the immediate popular support for such a move; they are also reasonably sure that there will be no opposition to such an allocation of resources. By contrast, a decision to embark on a public health policy in the form of alcohol controls would entail a long-term commitment to what might appear to be extremely moralistic ideals, in the certain knowledge that such policy will be immediately controversial and unpopular. This is not to say that researchers and organisations which draw on research findings are incapable of influencing the formulation of public policy, but rather that their success is dependent on gaining understanding of the policy process and working consistently to influence the key decision makers in the light of this understanding. Secker, on the basis of his experience, believes that lobbyists for the drinks industry are generally knowledgeable and adept when it comes to 'networking' ministers, their advisers and their civil servants. It is also important to point out, however, that the drinks industry has access to what can appear to be unlimited resources when it comes to funding its lobbying activities, while those who advocate the public health perspective usually operate within far more modest budgets.

In November 1986, INCA held a one-day conference with the title 'Alcohol, Preventing the Harm – Towards a National Policy', in line with the view expressed in *Planning for the Future* that INCA had a key role to play in the formulation of a national policy. Reading through the conference papers, it is relatively easy to see the battle lines which were being drawn but difficult to see how these differences could be reconciled. Dr Norman Kreitman, a British psychiatrist with considerable research experience in the alcohol field, argued trenchantly for a national alcohol policy which would reflect public health concerns; while Harry Hannon, representing the drinks industry, repudiated all suggestions that alcohol was a dangerous drug, arguing that 'The problem of abuse is a people problem, not a product problem'; and Liam Flanagan, Secretary of the Department of Health, discussed treatment services but gave no indication that his department was committed to playing a co-ordinating role in formulating a national policy which would reconcile all these conflicting interests.[42]

To some extent, this was to be INCA's last hurrah; the organisation which had been paralysed because of its own unresolved ideological tensions for almost fifteen years was now experiencing financial difficulties. It failed to negotiate a modest increase in the direct grant which it had been receiving from the Department of Health to supplement its income from the eight health boards, and in 1988 the Council voted to wind itself down. At the end of November 1988, INCA ceased operations; its National Director, Sally Edwards, worked on contract with the Health Promotion Unit for about six months following INCA's closure and one long-serving clerical worker moved into a permanent position with the Department of Health. The unwillingness of the Department of Health to provide the increase sought by INCA indicated that it was no longer – if it ever had been – greatly concerned to support this organisation, but it was an indirect and relatively passive action and it was not accompanied by any policy statement from the Department of Health clarifying or explaining its position on this issue. Utilising a health care metaphor, one could see the Department's behaviour as unplugging the life support machine rather than taking a more active role in terminating the life of a chronically ailing organisation. The Department of Health had played no part in setting up INCA, nor had it displayed initiative in any other area of alcohol policy; its indirect closure of INCA was, therefore, at least consistent with its track record in this area.

In seeking to understand why INCA closed at this point, the answer seems relatively straightforward from an internal organisational perspective. The various protagonists within INCA appear to have found it easier to capitulate and close down the organisation in the face of this new, albeit passive, hostility from the Department of Health than to mount a public campaign to stay open. While commercial sponsorship to stay open was potentially available, this might have involved accepting money from the drinks industry, which would have highlighted and widened the existing internal split. Perhaps what is more important, though less easy to discern, is the motivation of the Department of Health in effectively closing INCA. It will be recalled from Chapter One that health promotion ideas and ideals were being articulated explicitly for the first time in Ireland during these years. In 1986 the Department of Health had published *Health: The Wider Dimensions* which generally reflected the WHO vision of health promotion, and which specifically had decried the lack of a co-ordinated policy approach to alcohol and alcohol problems. In 1987 a similar document, *Promoting Health Through Public Policy,* was published by the Health Education Bureau, leading to the closure of the Bureau and the establishment within the Department of Health of a Health Promotion Unit.

One could surmise, therefore, that the simultaneous closure of the Health Education Bureau and INCA represented, as indeed the rhetoric of the period suggested, a coherent shift towards the realisation of these health promotion ideals. On the alcohol front, this could be seen as a demonstration of impatience with INCA and the beginning of a new era in which the Department of Health saw itself as leading the way in health promotion. Such a vision of the Department of Health taking a central role in building healthy public policy on alcohol would, of course, seem rather far-fetched in the light of its historic inactivity in this sphere, the most recent indicator of which was Liam Flanagan's pointed avoidance of commitment on this issue at the 1986 INCA conference.

Even though INCA had not been involved for many years in highly public advocacy or lobbying activities, its closure meant that there was now *no* independent lobby group with an interest in alcohol problems. Alcoholics Anonymous continued to flourish, but retained an interest only in individual problem drinkers and avoided any involvement with policy issues, in accordance with its traditions. It is worth noting that in the United Kingdom, where there had been no political welcome for healthy public policy on alcohol by the Thatcher Government, the DHSS had nonetheless taken the initiative in establishing a single, well-funded body, *Alcohol Concern,* which lobbied with a large degree of autonomy and professionalism in the face of strong opposition from the drinks industry.

Conclusion

The primary aim of this chapter was to describe the emergence internationally of the public health perspective and to explore how it was represented during the period 1973-1988 in the Irish health policy scene. It has shown that to all intents and purposes the public health perspective was diametrically opposed to the disease concept, involving a return to the point of view previously expressed in Ireland by the Intoxicating Liquor Commission of 1925. While this 'drier' policy perspective could claim to be based on a sounder scientific footing than previous attempts at alcohol control policies (which had tended more strongly towards a moral or temperance ethos) it was greatly hindered by the general cultural tolerance of alcohol and the specific view of alcohol problems which had grown up in the hey-day of the disease concept in post-war Ireland.

It was argued at the end of Chapter Two that the introduction of the disease concept to Ireland could be understood in policy terms as approximating to Lindblom's incremental model of policy making; within this framework the test of a good policy is not that it is demonstrably effective in a rational-technical sense or that it is consistent with public values, but simply that people like it. The major difficulty for proponents of the public health perspective was that it was generally unpalatable and appeared to have little hope of gaining widespread popularity. The decision to use the 'organisational network' approach to policy making – which involved a relatively elite group within INCA making approaches to political elites – was understandable and commendable from a public health point of view, but was ultimately of little value in view of the nature of the issues and the ambivalence and ineptitude of INCA itself.

However, with the demise of INCA the only potential source of policy change in the alcohol and health area appeared to be the newly-created Health Promotion Unit in the Department of Health, and it is the work of this unit on the task of formulating a national alcohol policy which will be the main topic of Chapter Four.

NOTES

1. J. Seeley, 'Alcoholism as a Disease: Implications for Social Policy', in D. Pittman and C. Snyder (eds), *Society, Culture and Drinking Patterns.* (New York: John Wiley, 1962), p.593.

2. N. Christie and K. Bruun, 'Alcohol Problems: The Conceptual Framework', in M. Keller and T. Coffey (eds), *Proceedings of the 28th International Congress on Alcohol and Alcoholism.* (Highland Park, New Jesey: Hillhouse Press, 1969) p.72.

3. Ibid, p.72.

4. D. Cahalan, *Problem Drinkers.* (San Francisco: Jossey-Bass, 1970); D. Cahalan and R. Room, *Problem Drinking Among American Men.* (New Brunswick, New Jersey: Rutger Centre of Alcohol Studies, 1974).

5. *The Lancet, 1* (1972), 'WHO and a New Perspective on Alcoholism', pp 1087-88.

6. J. Moser, 'What does an alcohol policy look like?' in I. Glass (ed.), *The International Handbook of Addiction Behaviour.* (London: Tavistock/ Routledge, 1991), pp. 313-319.

7. J. Orford and G. Edwards, *Alcoholism: A Comparison of Treatment and Advice, with a Study of the Influence of Marriage. (*Oxford University Press, 1977).

8. G. Vaillant, *The Natural History of Alcoholism.* (Harvard University Press, 1983), p.284.

9. S. Peele, *Diseasing of America: Addiction Treatment out of Control.* (Lexington, Mass.: Lexington Books, 1989).

10. *Appendix A, Report to the Minister for Health by the Irish National Council on Alcoholism (*January 1973).

11. Ibid., p.49.

12. Ibid., p.49.

13. Ibid., p.50.

14. Ibid., p.51.

15. National Economic and Social Council, *Health Services: The Implications of Demographic Change (*NESC Paper No. 73) (Dublin: NESC, 1983), p.46.

16. A. O'Hare and D. Walsh, *Activities of Irish Psychiatric Hospitals and Units 1979.* (Dublin: Medico-Social Research Board, 1981).

17. This statement of Dr Stevenson's views are based on numerous discussions with him over a period of six years (1977-1983) during which time this writer worked with Dr Stevenson at St Dymphna's Hospital in Dublin.

18. The growing support of the Medico-Social Research Board (MSRB) for the public health perspective is discernible in its annual reports throughout the 1970s. Another publication which specifically confirms this swing towards the public health approach resulted from a collaborative project involving Dermot Walsh of the MSRB and Phil Davies of the Department of Medical Sociology at the University of Aberdeen: P. Davies and D. Walsh, *Alcohol Problems and Alcohol Control in Europe.* (London: Croom Helm, 1983).

19. *Appendix B, Report to the Minister for Health by the Irish National Council on Alcoholism* (January 1973).

20. D. Walsh and B. Walsh, 'Drowning the Shamrock: Alcohol and Drink in Ireland' in E. Single et al, *Alcohol, Society and the State* (Vol. 2): *The Social History of*

Control Policy in Seven Countries. (Toronto: Addiction Research Foundation, 1981), p.120.

21. D. Anderson, *Perspectives on Treatment: The Minnesota Experience.* (Center City, Minnesota: Hazelden, 1981).

22. Ibid, p.7 (It should be pointed out that the 'recovery rate' claimed here has never been substantiated by evaluative research published in peer reviewed journals.

23. Minutes of Eastern Health Board Meeting of 12 January, 1978.

24. Ibid.

25. Letter (26 January, 1978) from Fr Raphael Short to all members of the Eastern Health Board – given to this writer by Noreen Kearney, a board member at that time.

26. *The Psychiatric Services: Planning for the Future.* (Dublin: Stationery Office, 1984), chapter 13.

27. Information from VHI Annual Reports, supplemented by additional data given to this writer by VHI's research department.

28. *The Irish Press,* 22 March, 1985.

29. Letter to *Irish Times,* 2 April, 1985.

30. Minutes of Meeting of the Irish National Council on Alcoholism, 14 September, 1984.

31. Minutes of Meeting of the Irish National Council on Alcoholism, 10 April, 1985.

32. *The Psychiatric Services: Planning for the Future,* cit. sup., pp 112-113.

33. INCA Submission to the Minister for Health (1979), p.1.

34. *Availability Control Policy – Consumption of Alcohol* (INCA submission to the Minister for Justice, 1980), p.6.

35. R.D. Stevenson, personal communication (undated but written almost certainly in 1986).

36. Minutes of the Meeting of the Irish National Council on Alcoholism held on 14 September, 1984.

37. Report on Meeting with Mr Gordon Grimm, Senior Executive and Director of Education and Training, Hazelden, and with Ms Marilyn Brisett, Director of Counsellor Training, Hazelden; 18 June 1984 (Circulated to Members of INCA's Executive Committee for Meeting of 22 June 1984).

38. *Joint Oireachtas Committee on Legislation; Review of Licensing Laws: Minutes of Evidence of Oral Submissions, 24 September, 1985,* p.30.

39. Ibid., p.27.

40. The following reports published by the Drinks Industry Group: *The Economic Importance of the Drinks Industry in Ireland* (1982); *The Taxation of Alcoholic Beverages in Ireland* (1983); *A Summary of Retailers of Alcohol in Ireland* (1983); *The Drinks Industry in Ireland* (1986).

41. A. Secker, 'The policy-research interface: an insider's view', *Addiction,* 88 (Supplement), (1993), pp 115-116S.

42. *Proceedings of INCA Conference, Alcoholism. Preventing the Harm: Towards a National Policy (*November 27, 1986).

◆ 4

Formulating a National Alcohol Policy 1988-1996

Introduction

Commencing with the establishment of a Health Promotion Unit within the Department of Health in 1988, a broader framework for the implementation of health promotion policy in Ireland was created over the next few years. Amongst the structures established at this time were an Advisory Council on Health Promotion which was meant to monitor and assist in the work of the HPU; in political terms, the most important element in this framework was the decision to set up a Cabinet Sub-Committee on Health Promotion and, in academic and scientific terms, the funding of a new Chair of Health Promotion at University College Galway was particularly significant.[1] The creation of these core health promotion structures generally suggested that health promotion was now set to become a reality and, for those interested in alcohol issues, there was the added bonus that policy making in relation to alcohol was identified as being particularly suited to the health promotional perspective.

This chapter will therefore examine policy developments between 1988 and 1996, the period in which health promotion concepts were most explicitly applied to alcohol policy and when expectations on this issue were most raised.

The Intoxicating Liquor Act, 1988

Before embarking on a detailed account of how the Health Promotion Unit (HPU) tackled the formidable task of drafting a national alcohol policy, it is necessary to have a brief discussion of the Intoxicating Liquor Act, 1988, since this will shed additional light on the policy climate within which the HPU was operating.

The 1988 legislation had been in the offing for several years: the 1984 planning document *Building on Reality* initially proposed the granting of full liquor licences to restaurants; the Joint Oireachtas Committee on Legislation had considered the licensing laws in 1985; and an Intoxicating Liquor Bill, 1986 had lapsed with the dissolution of the twenty-fourth Dáil in early 1987. In early 1988, Deputy Seán Barrett of Fine Gael introduced a Private Member's Bill known as the Intoxicating Liquor (Children and Young Persons) Bill. This bill was received with general sympathy from all sides of the Dáil but ultimately failed to get support because the Minister for Justice, Gerry Collins, made it clear that his own bill was now ready for the legislative process.

The rationale underlying this Fianna Fáil bill, known simply as the Intoxicating Liquor Bill, 1988, was presented in detail by Mr Collins at the beginning of the Second Stage debate in Dáil Éireann on 26 April, 1988. The difficulties and – from a health promotion perspective – the contradictions inherent in this legislation are evident from the Minister's opening remarks:

> There are a number of reasons for bringing forward this important Bill. Its most important objective is to help curb drink abuse, particularly as far as under-age drinking is concerned. At the same time, to meet public demand in relation to certain aspects of the legislation, the Bill makes some adjustments in the prohibited hours and proposes that special provisions be made to enable restaurants of an acceptable standard to serve a full range of alcoholic drinks.[2]

What the Minister was proposing was to continue generally with the liberalising trend in the licensing system which had commenced in 1960, while at the same time hoping to curb 'drink abuse' through the introduction of some specific amendments in relation to under-age drinking. The logic of this legislative proposal was much closer to that of the disease concept than to that of the public health perspective; the implication was that increasing the number of retail outlets and extending the hours during which alcohol could be legally purchased would not necessarily affect the incidence and prevalence of alcohol-related problems. The public health perspective, on the other hand, did not view problem drinking as categorically different from 'social' drinking and tended to the view that policy aimed at reducing the incidence and prevalence of problems could only succeed when it was aimed at the totality of societal drinking behaviours. The 1988 bill proposed specifically to:

- allow approved restaurants full liquor licences without the necessity of 'extinguishing' existing licences (Sections 5–24)
- extend the opening hours on Sundays till 11.00pm (Section 25)
- extend the 'drinking-up' period from ten minutes to half an hour, thereby effectively allowing pubs to remain open till 11.30pm in winter and 12.00 midnight in summer (Section 27)

- abolish the 'holy hour', the mandatory closing period from 2.30pm to 3.30pm, in Cork and Dublin (Section 25).

One of the main measures to prevent problems amongst under-age drinkers was contained in a proposal to omit the word 'knowingly' from Section 31 of the new legislation which made it an offence for retailers to sell drink to those under the age of eighteen; the existing legislation was regarded as difficult to enforce since it could not readily be proven that a publican had 'knowingly' sold drink to an under-age customer. It was also proposed to make it an offence for those under the age of eighteen to purchase alcohol (Section 33), and to allow the Gardaí to confiscate alcoholic drinks from under-age drinkers if they were in possession of such drinks in a public place (Section 37). The legislation made provision for a voluntary 'age card' scheme which would assist publicans in determining the age of customers who might be under-age (Section 40). On balance, however, it would have to be concluded that the Intoxicating Liquor Bill, 1988 concentrated on young drinkers as though they primarily were involved in problem drinking, while the general thrust of the legislation was to make alcohol more accessible to adult drinkers. In terms of the public health perspective – which argued for policy dealing with societal alcohol consumption as a whole – the bill was inherently contradictory, if not downright hypocritical.

The Dáil and Seanad debates on this legislation contain no reference to public health or health promotion and there is no indication that politicians had been lobbied from such a perspective. Deputy Seán Barrett, who had earlier introduced his own Private Member's Bill on this subject, did admittedly argue that 'If we are serious about dealing with alcohol abuse, surely the minimum we should do is to fund to a reasonable extent such important bodies as the Irish National Council on Alcohol'.[3] On the whole, however, there was a large measure of consensus across parties that the Minister had done well on this complex policy issue; the independent, NUI Senator, John A. Murphy, exemplified this view when he considered the bill from an historical perspective, concluding: 'Anyway, in the whole context, the State has done well in its public policy on drink, a sensible and balanced policy on the whole, I think'.[4]

While there was no evidence that politicians had been lobbied by representatives of the health sector, it was abundantly clear that intensive lobbying had been done by two competing interest groups, the restaurateurs and hoteliers who were eager to be given full liquor licences and the existing vintners who were strongly opposed to this development. The vintners' argument reflected the fact that they had traditionally enjoyed a monopoly on the sale of alcoholic drinks for consumption 'on the premises' and that they were reluctant to see this monopoly ended by the granting of special restaurant licences. On this occasion, the vintners were less concerned with presenting a libertarian defence of the right of adults to have ready access to alcohol than they were with portraying themselves as guardians of public health and public order. Their contention was that granting new licences to restaurateurs not only gave an unfair advantage to the restaurateurs, but also was likely to be uncontrollable when all food outlets became *de facto* bars. In the Seanad, for example, Senator Tom McEllistrim addressed himself as follows to the Minister for Justice:

> It has also been mentioned to me – and I would like the Minister to give me an assurance on this – that fish and chip shops will get a licence eventually. That has been claimed by some publicans.[5]

Deputy Michael McDowell, during the Dáil debate, spoke of the monopoly value of the existing licences and the investment which vintners had made in these licences, although ultimately arguing that 'The licensing laws were not designed to create monopoly rights for anybody'.[6] The Minister, Gerry Collins, had also been quite open and explicit about the difficulties involved in legislating in an area of competing sectional interests which, as he put it, could degenerate into 'an unmerciful tug-of-war'.[7]

The Minister's legislative proposals were enacted without substantial change, and the granting of special restaurant licences was arranged in a way that reflected what might be considered a customary political compromise between conflicting interests. Restaurateurs who had argued for full liquor licences for their premises were placated in the sense that this was now legally permissible, while the vintners were placated by the stringent conditions attaching to these new licences. Restaurants could only apply for a licence when they conformed to high catering and accommodation standards which were certified by Bord Fáilte; they had to have a waiting area which was not a bar; drink could only be served to a person for whom a substantial meal was ordered, and the once-off licence fee was £3,000. The spectre of fish and chip shops and other fast-food outlets selling drink around the clock amidst scenes of wild abandon had been well and truly laid to rest.

Section 47 of the Intoxicating Liquor Act, 1988 was, on the face of it, the only section of this new legislation which reflected health promotion principles: it prohibited supermarkets and self-service groceries from displaying alcoholic beverages alongside food-stuffs, and was intended to stop impulse buying of drink and to introduce greater control over purchases than could reasonably be expected at busy checkouts. It restricted the sale of alcohol in supermarkets to special intoxicating liquor counters and, in its own modest way, could be compared to the system of state monopoly outlets in countries which had a strong temperance tradition and which wished to demonstrate through their sales' systems that alcohol, though licit, was a 'demerit' good. Section 47, however, has never been brought into operation by the Minister for Justice and there has been no indication that this situation is likely to change.

While there were increases in the numbers of successful prosecutions for sale of alcohol to under-age drinkers following the 1988 legislation, research into the prevalence of under-age drinking suggested that this behaviour had increased to the point where it was now normative rather than deviant. Morgan and Grube (1994) surveyed drinking behaviour amongst Dublin post-primary school pupils during 1991 and found evidence of dramatic increases in drinking since a comparable survey which they had conducted eight years earlier. For example, of their total sample – which extended across the range of post-primary ages from twelve to nineteen – four-fifths of the pupils had consumed alcohol at some time as opposed to two-thirds eight years earlier. Abstainers at the age of 17 now made up only seven per cent of this age-group as opposed to twenty-one per cent eight years earlier. These researchers did not offer definitive explanations as to why young people were drinking at an earlier age than previously, but suggested that one causal factor was the change in the normative climate surrounding alcohol. In comparison to the earlier survey, young people now thought that there was relatively less disapproval of their drinking both by parents and peers and that, in fact, parents and peers were now more likely to approve of their drinking.[8]

If one takes the parliamentary debate and the wider political activity surrounding the enactment of the Intoxicating Liquor Act, 1988 as a measure of the policy climate in which the HPU was about to begin its work on the formulation of a national alcohol policy, then it is clear that the HPU could scarcely be confronted with a more indifferent – if not hostile – environment within which to achieve its health promotional aims.

The Health Promotion Unit and the national alcohol policy

Following the closure of INCA in 1988, its last director, Sally Edwards, worked on contract with the HPU for a period of about six months, during which time she did some preliminary work on the possibility of formulating a national alcohol policy. However, it was to be some time later before the task of drafting such a policy became part of the official agenda of the HPU. During 1990, the Minister for Health formally requested the Advisory Council on Health Promotion to take on this task, with the HPU acting as its resource body for research, secretarial and general support. The Advisory Council had been hindered by the sudden death of its first Chairperson, Dr Ivo Drury, in 1989, but following his replacement in 1990, work began on the national alcohol policy. In February 1991, advertisements were placed in the newspapers describing the task being undertaken by the Advisory Council on Health Promotion and inviting interested parties to make written submissions. The public notice, in part, read as follows:

> The Government has decided that a National Alcohol Policy should be formulated. In pursuance of that decision, the Minister for Health has requested the Advisory Council on Health Promotion to develop a broadly based policy, and to make recommendations to him for presentation to Government.
>
> The Council is examining alcohol, its availability, consumption, use and abuse under broad headings including historical, social, cultural, economic and legal factors, together with such matters as education, advertising, prevention, diagnosis and treatment strategies, etc., and particularly the issues of youth and alcohol, and the role of parents and family ...[9]

There was in the style of this notice a definite suggestion of the rational comprehensive approach to policy making, at least insofar as it related to the work of the Advisory Council on Health Promotion. The implication was that the Advisory Council was embarking on a root and branch assessment of all aspects of alcohol production, importation, retailing and consumption in Ireland; research findings would be sought and utilised, and the draft policy submitted to the Minister would represent a rational attempt at maximising health.

Within a short period of the beginning of this process, two events occurred which effectively transferred control of alcohol-policy affairs from the Advisory Council to the HPU. By a sad coincidence, the new Chairperson of the Advisory Council, Dr Ciarán Barry, died in early 1991 just as submissions on the national alcohol policy were coming in from interested individuals and institutions. He was not replaced until late 1992 when Frances Fitzgerald, a social worker who had been an activist in the Women's Political Association, was appointed to the position; within weeks of her appointment, Frances Fitzgerald was elected to Dáil Éireann as a Fine Gael deputy and this new party political role necessitated her resignation from the Advisory Council on Health Promotion. She was never replaced, and in the absence of an independent Chairperson – effectively from 1991 to the end of the period studied in 1996 – responsibility, as well as a large measure of power and influence, within the health promotion structure devolved to the staff of the HPU.

The second event which strengthened the hand of the civil service in the formulation of a national alcohol policy was the decision taken in May

1991 to establish a separate Working Group to concentrate on this task. Of the sixteen surviving, non-civil service members of the Advisory Council, only three were retained on this new Working Group while six other people, who were thought to have specific experience and expertise in the field of alcohol, were co-opted for this task.[10] This decision was reasonable, since the 'broadly based'[11] Advisory Council could not be expected to have specific expertise in the field of alcohol; however, the *ad hoc* status of this Working Group and the fact that it was chaired by the Principal Officer of the HPU rather than by an independent outsider was to have a major influence on the pace and style of its deliberations.

As described in Chapters Two and Three, the Department of Health had previously displayed no initiative in relation to alcohol policy; in particular, it should be recalled that in 1986, when addressing INCA's conference on the then hypothetical question of a national alcohol policy, Liam Flanagan (Secretary of the Department of Health) had expressed no enthusiasm for or commitment to such a project. The decision to commit the Advisory Council and the HPU to the business of drafting the policy had been that of Dr Rory O'Hanlon, Minister for Health from 1987 to 1992 and architect of the new health promotion structure.

The new Working Group met for the first time in June 1991, by which time about 150 written submissions had been received and a number of commissioned reports from the Economic and Social Research Institute (ESRI) had been completed. These ESRI reports did not make easy reading for those in favour of the public health perspective; they were compiled by two economists, Denis Coniffe and Danny McCoy, and their overall conclusions were broadly similar to those contained in the commissioned reports of the Drinks Industry Group. In summary, they argued:

- that the drinks industry was of major importance to the Irish economy in terms of revenue, job creation and exports
- that Irish alcohol consumption rates were modest by international standards
- that the perceived commitment of Irish people to alcohol consumption, as measured by the proportion of gross disposable income spent on alcohol, had previously been exaggerated by the failure to understand differences in the accounting conventions used in international comparisons
- that alcohol consumption in Ireland was much more sensitive to income than to price, and, in any event, that Ireland's already expensive alcohol could not readily be made more expensive in the context of tax harmonisation within the Single Market of the European Union.

The Working Group had the opportunity to meet the authors of these ESRI reports, but this meeting served mainly to confirm that the economists had little sympathy for the WHO's preferred strategy for the reduction of alcohol-related problems. A further paper which reviewed Irish drinking habits from an anthropological perspective was subsequently commissioned, to some extent as an antidote to the views of the economists, but this took some time and ultimately made little impact on the Working Group.[12]

The Working Group was now chaired by the Principal Officer of the HPU, a civil servant who – in the generalist tradition of the Irish civil service – could expect to spend at most four to five years in this section before being transferred back to more mainstream curative concerns and functions in the Department of Health. The task facing the Principal Officer in relation to the formulation of a national alcohol policy was, by any standard, a difficult one. Irish alcohol policy, at this time in the early 1990s, still largely reflected the tenets of the disease concept and was the end result of a process of incremental drift which had taken place since the end of World War II. Now, however, the idea of an immediate and radical policy change had been put on the agenda, and expectations had been raised on this score by the Minister's public announcement of his decision to draft a national alcohol policy. The expectations of health promotionists were of a return to a 'drier' policy perspective with various alcohol control strategies being utilised to reduce consumption. The preliminary work by the HPU and the Advisory Council had merely served, however, to illustrate how polarised this policy situation was. Those who were familiar with or sympathetic towards the public health perspective on alcohol were few in number, even perhaps in the Department of Health itself, and the task of the HPU appeared to be that of co-ordinating this small group so as to make the maximum impact in this area.

Of the three policy models discussed in Chapter One, it would seem that *partisan mutual adjustment*, of a passive and incremental style, corresponds most closely to the way in which the HPU handled the task of formulating a national alcohol policy; the concept of *nondecision-making* in public policy-making, which was devised by Bachrach and Baratz (1963; 1970), also has some application and this will now be considered here. This concept was used to argue that power in the policy-making sphere does not solely consist of the overt process of influencing events so that one policy option is favoured rather than another; nondecision-making refers to power which is exerted in more subtle, covert ways to ensure that particularly contentious issues or debates are kept off the policy-making agenda. One could surmise that, given their long history of inactivity in this field, senior civil servants in the Department of Health would have preferred to avoid becoming embroiled in policy debate in which the public health perspective was pitted against the disease concept. However, the Minister's enthusiasm for his newly-created health promotion structures and his determination to tackle alcohol problems from this perspective appeared to spell an end to the nondecision-making era. Like it or not, the HPU was now expected to play a central role in tackling these difficult policy issues and in drafting definite policy proposals for submission to Government. The tactics employed by the HPU in responding to this challenge will now be described; generally it will be argued that in overall terms these tactics constitute an extension of nondecision-making in the sense that they protracted the decision-making process, successfully prevented the issues from becoming publicly contentious, and, while creating an impression of openness and consultation, served to retain control of policy-making within the civil service structure of the HPU.

Between June 1991 and March 1992, the Working Group met delegations from some of the organisations which had already made written submissions; the organisations selected for participation in this formal consultation process were those deemed to be most influential. This consultation process, which is commonplace in public policy-making, appeared in this instance to be largely ritualistic and wasteful of time; in the experience of this writer, none of the groups consulted in this way made any additional points in their oral submissions, and generally they did not present their arguments as clearly or as effectively at these meetings as they had done on paper.

In March 1992, the Chairman of the Working Group wrote to its members suggesting that the best way to 'develop the direction and content of the Report' was to look at policy options in the light of working papers on about half a dozen topics to be drafted by the HPU.[13] Between March and September 1992, these working papers were drafted and circulated to members, but only two meetings of the Working Group took place. In February 1993, following an inquiry from this writer as to whether the Working Group would meet and finish its task, the Chairman replied as follows:

> Following receipt of the observations of each of the members of the Working Group a draft comprehensive report on this Policy was prepared by the Health Promotion Unit which reflected, to the greatest extent possible, the various views expressed by the members.
>
> The draft Report was then circulated to members of the Advisory Council on Health Promotion and was to be considered at their subsequent meeting scheduled for November. However, this subsequent meeting of the Council had to be postponed for reasons beyond the control of the Unit. We are in the process

of convening another meeting of the Advisory Council to consider the draft Report following which we propose submitting it to the Minister.[14]

A request by this writer to be sent a copy of the draft report went unanswered.

For the fifteen months when it had ostensibly been an active body, the Working Group had done nothing other than meet delegations from various interest groups and read background literature on this thorny policy issue. Now, at a point when it might be expected to tackle the subject, the Chairman simply stopped convening meetings, without informing members that no further meetings would take place or that a document which purported to reflect their views had been drawn up by the HPU. This latter document was not signed by the members of the Working Group and was not made available to the six members who had been co-opted, although it was presumably circulated to the four members who had come from the Advisory Council.

Despite the optimism expressed by the Chairman (in the letter cited above) that a national alcohol policy would be quickly drafted and sent for Government approval, this process was not completed until September 1996, some three and a half years later. Over these years, references to the national policy cropped up in various health policy documents without any explanation as to why this delay was taking place or what the difficulties were. As early as 1992, the *Green Paper on Mental Health* had described the multi-sectoral nature of the health promotion approach to alcohol problems and indicated that: 'The Council is well advanced with its task'.[15] Two years later, however, in May 1994, *Shaping a Healthier Future,* Minister Brendan Howlin's healthcare strategy for the remainder of the decade, identified the necessity to promote moderation in alcohol consumption as one of its targets; the rhetoric was now somewhat more restrained and less radical in its view of health promotion in this sphere and, without going into detail, promised 'A national policy on alcohol which will be adopted and launched during the next twelve months'.[16] The entire health promotion concept and Irish health promotion structures were the subject of yet another policy document, *A Health Promotion Strategy: Making the Healthier Choice the Easier Choice,* published by the HPU in July 1995. This contained only a brief reference to:

> The development of a national policy to promote moderation in alcohol consumption and reduce risks to physical, mental and family health associated with alcohol misuse – such policy to be adopted and launched during 1995.[17]

Some of its members remained under the impression that the Working Group would be reconvened, since it seemed unlikely that the HPU would present a report ostensibly representing collective views without first clearing the draft report with the group. In fact the group was never reconvened, and the first time that most members saw the national alcohol policy document was following its publication in September 1996, some four years after the Working Group had last met. During this protracted gestation period, surprise or disquiet was expressed from time to time by interested parties at what was seen as an inordinate delay in completing this task. An editorial in the *Irish Medical Times* during October 1995, for example, castigated the Department of Health for its delay in publishing a policy document on 'alcoholism'; this paper had been told that the policy document would be published within the next few months, a promise which was received with scepticism because 'there has already been evidence that the Department is being particularly slow to meet this issue head on'.[18] From a policy analysis point of view, this latter comment is probably a good deal more revealing than its author intended. It is not part of the culture of the Irish civil service to tackle issues 'head on', where this implies the espousal and single-minded promotion of a policy line which is deemed to be socially worthy but which lacks popular and political support. While the foregoing account of the handling of the national alcohol policy issue by the HPU clearly suggests a continuance of nondecision-making, it is important to attempt to understand the motivation of the HPU in dragging its heels on this matter. It has commonly been suggested that senior civil servants in Ireland have been characterised by rigidity, secrecy and conservatism, and that they have found it easier to administer existing policy than to play an imaginative role in devising new policy. Policy analysts have also argued that Government Ministers come and go with great regularity and that they vary greatly in terms of their competence in and commitment to the ministries to which they are appointed, and, in these circumstances, it is understandable that senior civil servants – sometimes referred to sardonically as the 'permanent government' – wield a good deal more policy-making influence than is officially theirs under the legal convention of *corporation sole*.

The Minister for Health who charged the Advisory Council on Health Promotion with the task of drafting a national alcohol policy in 1990 was Dr Rory O'Hanlon; however, by the time this policy document was agreed by Government and publicly launched in September 1996, the following had all served for varying periods of time as Minister for Health: Dr John O'Connell, Mary O'Rourke, Brendan Howlin and Michael Noonan. None of these subsequent Ministers rescinded the decision to develop a national alcohol policy, yet neither did it appear to be a political priority for any of them. It seems reasonable to assume that the staff of the HPU detected little or no evidence of serious political commitment on the part of successive ministers to the radical style of health promotion which would have been necessary in order to make healthy public policy a reality in the alcohol sphere; furthermore, even if there had been a minister with a philosophical commitment to alcohol control policies, it must have been equally apparent that other ministers would not readily subordinate their own sectoral interest to the overall health interest.

It seems clear that the Department of Health had been reluctant in the first instance to have the notion of a comprehensive national alcohol policy dominated by the health interest placed on the public policy agenda. However, having had this task imposed upon it by an enthusiastic Minister, it confirmed its impossibility in terms of *realpolitik* and, in order to avoid divisive public debate and the embarrassment of revealing serious flaws in the entire health promotion edifice, opted for a protracted policy-making process. Indeed, there is reason to believe that left to its own devices the HPU would have deferred the launch of the national alcohol policy even further; the Minister for Health, Michael Noonan, appears to have decided that it was timely to launch the national policy in September 1996, perhaps because during this month the Dáil Select Committee on Legislation and Security was holding hearings on the licensing laws and was considering a further extension of the opening hours. There had been no public health contribution to the debate on the Intoxicating Liquor Act, 1988, and with all policy matters in abeyance till the national policy was launched, a similar gap in the debate could easily have occurred again on this occasion. The strongest evidence that the launch of the national policy was a Ministerial decision, imposed upon the HPU, is to be found in the fact that at the public launch of the policy on 19 September, 1996 – having been in preparation for almost six years – there was still no published policy document; instead, the media were supplied with what appeared to be a hastily-prepared Executive Summary and it was made known that this was an advance copy and that the full policy document and summary were 'with the printers'.

The full report which was published a few weeks after the official launch was, as was customary for health promotion documents, presented and packaged in a most attractive style. The report was entitled *National Alcohol Policy – Ireland*[19] and consisted of three main sections. Section 1 set the context for the national alcohol policy by reviewing alcohol consumption trends in Ireland: it compared the Irish drinking experience with the experience of other countries, summarised the data on alcohol problems, and finally looked at the positive aspects of alcohol consumption – including the economic role of alcohol in Ireland. Section 2 then introduced and described the public health perspective on alcohol before going on to review a range of *individual* and *environmental* strategies which could be utilised in pursuit of public health objectives in this area. Sections 1 and 2 were well written and authoritative, but Section 3 which presented a 'Plan of Action' was from a health promotional point of view both the most important and the most disappointing element of the report. This final section was couched in the language of strategic management, referring to target groups and target settings, all in the context of the role which non-governmental agencies and Government departments other than Health had to play in the implementation of the policy. However, a close reading of this Plan of Action makes it clear that, in the process of compiling the report, the HPU had not succeeded in making fruitful strategic alliances with other sectors of Government, with the drinks industry or with community groupings so as to maximise the prospects for real health promotion in relation to alcohol. Section 3 was characterised throughout by the vagueness and aspirational quality of its language, which was primarily about traditional attempts at 'encouraging' and 'making aware', and contained absolutely no suggestion of new alcohol controls being introduced as part of a healthy public policy initiative. Any fears that the drinks industry might have felt about the new national alcohol policy being a form of neo-Prohibitionism must surely have been dispelled by a quick reading of this report, since it could not in truth be said that there was even a single concrete proposal contained therein which was substantially different to anything that had previously been tried.

Newspaper accounts of the launch of the national alcohol policy also suggest that the Minister for Health was ambivalent and generally uncomfortable with the whole subject of alcohol controls. He told reporters that he 'would be telling the Select Dáil Committee on Legislation and Security, which was currently reviewing the licensing laws, that he was opposed to any extension of hours'.[20] On the other hand, when it was suggested to him by journalists that the policy might have been tougher and that it lacked 'teeth', he revealed his unease with the paternalism inherent in alcohol control policies; his reply was:

> It's very hard to legislate for virtue. It's even difficult enough to legislate for good behaviour. The kind of island I would like to see is where we would have what I would describe as sovereign individuals who are well-educated and mature and that when you give them information which is relevant to their own well-being they will make individual sovereign decisions in their own interest. I think that's the best approach.[21]

In concluding this account of the launch of the national alcohol policy, it is important to point out that it was not merely the vagueness and aspirational quality of its content which might have made it seem unconvincing to those who might have hoped for a more incisive policy; what was equally discouraging was that the implementation of its plan of action was reliant on the co-operation of partners from other sectors of Government – co-operation which had not previously been forthcoming – while the overall monitoring of its implementation seemed set to remain with the HPU.

The failure of the HPU to deliver a co-ordinated national alcohol policy along health promotional lines was largely predictable; the debate which surrounded the Intoxicating Liquor Act, 1988 had made it clear that the policy climate remained inimical to the aspirations of public health activists. What emerged from this lengthy period of policy formulation is almost certainly best described in terms of the models of policy co-ordination outlined in Chapter One, as *partisan mutual adjustment.* It was a policy compromise in which all interested parties had to adjust their expectations and settle for something less than what they might have regarded as the optimum policy outcome. The Drinks Industry Group (DIG) would undoubtedly have preferred a policy document which reiterated what it saw as the simple truths of the disease concept, namely that their product was a perfectly safe one and that it was unfortunate that there were some 'bad' or defective consumers; nonetheless, the DIG must have been happy with the eventual policy document which rehearsed all their usual arguments about the economic significance of the industry, while at the same time acknowledging the protective role of alcohol in reducing the risk of coronary heart disease. Public health activists, on the other hand, must surely have felt disappointment that the concept of an integrated governmental alcohol policy based upon health principles, did not emerge from this lengthy process, while at the same time welcoming its commitment to enhanced alcohol awareness programmes. The main question which emerges from a consideration of this process of bargaining and compromise is whether the public health perspective could have been represented better: could the HPU have negotiated along the lines of the policy co-ordination model described by Harrison and Tether as *organisational networks,* or if it had failed to do so up to the launch of the national alcohol policy, had it the potential to develop this approach to policy making? These are the questions which will be addressed in the following section.

The Health Promotion Unit as an organisational networker?

It will be recalled from Chapter One that in their review of policy-making models for the co-ordination of alcohol and drug policy, Harrison and Tether concluded that the likelihood of achieving a rational-comprehensive or a corporate model, in which health was the dominant policy objective to which all other departmental or sectoral interests were subordinated, was negligible. They were critical of partisan mutual adjustment, not because they saw it as an inaccurate account of the reality of policy making in this area, but because in terms of public health values they deemed it to be excessively *laissez faire*.

Prescriptively, Harrison and Tether went on to recommend a third policy co-ordination approach – and one which has become increasingly popular in the meantime – namely the organisational networks model. This, in many ways, was a compromise between the other two models in that it accepted that the rational-comprehensive model was utopian, but argued that the health interest could be tactically pursued through a relatively loose framework or *network* of organisations, and that the results of such a process would be greater than those which could be achieved through the more informal system of partisan mutual adjustment. They also argued that in many instances such a network would consist of sections or sub-units of large organisations rather than whole organisations. It was suggested that sometimes such sub-units were at the periphery of their parent organisation and might have more in common with sub-units of other organisations than with their parent organisation. It could, for instance, be argued that in relation to alcohol problems among young people, the HPU had more in common with the Psychological Service of the Department of Education, or the Juvenile Liaison Section of the Garda Síochána or the Probation and Welfare Service of the Department of Justice than with the rest of the Department of Health.

The question which Harrison and Tether's concept of organisational networks raises is whether the HPU has the capacity to either play a central role – the spider at the centre of the web, as it were – or even to participate actively as an equal partner in such a network. Before looking critically at this question, it is useful to recall the five key elements of the Ottawa Charter on Health Promotion (set out in Chapter One) and to consider their application to Irish alcohol policy. These elements are:

- building healthy public policy
- creating supportive environments
- strengthening community action
- developing personal skills
- reorienting health services.

The final document, *The National Alcohol Policy: Ireland*, must be seen as effectively acknowledging the impossibility of realising the first of these elements, healthy public policy, in the alcohol sphere; the notion that other sectors of government would defer to the health interest proved to be illusory and, despite some residual references to multi-sectoral cooperation, it was clear that there was to be no unified and authoritative national alcohol policy aimed at promoting health. In fairness to the HPU, it could not really be said that any country had achieved the goal of healthy public policy in the alcohol domain as originally envisaged by the WHO, and indeed the WHO itself in its *European Charter on Alcohol* (drawn up in December 1995) had greatly moderated its tone in this regard. The last of the Ottawa Charter elements, reorienting health services, will be considered in the next section, but it is the middle three – creating supportive environments, strengthening community action and developing personal skills – which will now be considered in the context of the HPU's networking capacity.

National Alcohol Policy: Ireland accepted, albeit tacitly, that there could be no authoritative top-down policy which would effectively control alcohol availability and consumption in Ireland. The task of the HPU in relation to the development of life skills, the creation of supportive environments and the fostering of community action may be regarded, therefore, as a facilitative one, generally aimed at changing communal attitudes to alcohol as well as actual drinking behaviours. The evidence summarised in the completed policy document clearly demonstrated that alcohol had become increasingly normalised in Ireland, regarded, that is, as a relatively safe commodity which featured in various ways in everyday life. For example, the summary of the economic arguments about price and income elasticities confirmed that Irish consumption was in overall terms price inelastic, and that at most all that could be achieved through pricing was some degree of switching to low alcohol drinks; on the other hand, Irish alcohol consumption is generally income elastic, suggesting that economic growth is likely to lead to a disproportionate increase in consumption.[22] One other statistic which clearly illustrates the increased prominence and availability of alcohol in Irish social life is that referring to special exemption orders, the granting of extensions of opening hours for special occasions: in 1967 the courts had granted 6,342 of these orders, but by 1994 this had increased to 55,290.[23] Finally, in this context, the national alcohol policy document referred to the pervasiveness of alcohol advertising and to the promotion of sporting, social and cultural events by the drinks industry; it did not, however, refer specifically to the controversial sponsorship of the Gaelic Athletic Association's (GAA) All-Ireland Hurling Championship by Guinness Ireland.

Generally, it has to be concluded that the HPU displayed little interest in or aptitude for alcohol policy-making based on networking. Instead, it worked at a very slow pace on this project, controlling events rather than fostering alliances, and taking no risks when issues seemed contentious or controversial. The organisational networks model, as already described, is dependent on a peripheral sub-unit within a large organisation displaying a willingness to pursue common policy goals through collaboration with other peripheral sub-units or other interest groups outside its parent organisation. In the case of the HPU and its policy-making activity in the alcohol sphere, this might, for example, involve the Unit in forming a strategic alliance with: self-regulating bodies such as the Advertising Standards Authority of Ireland; professional bodies such as the Irish College of General Practitioners or the Irish Association of Alcohol and Addiction Counsellors; specific lobby groups such as Mothers Against Drink Driving; trade associations such as the Licensed Vintners Association, and many other relevant groups. The style of negotiation implied by this model is a style which is characterised by boldness, initiative and some degree of risk-taking, rather than by timidity and caution – where the peripheral sub-unit is constantly looking over its shoulder lest it incur the wrath of the parent organisation.

The HPU is, however, just one section of the Department of Health and civil servants who work in this unit, in keeping with the tradition of generalism in the Irish civil service, can expect to spend just a few years there before being transferred back to more mainstream departmental duties. There is, therefore, no real incentive for civil servants posted to the HPU to develop a passionate commitment to reducing alcohol-related problems or to any other aspect of health promotion; indeed, one could argue that passion and risk-taking of this kind would be viewed with considerable suspicion by colleagues and superiors, and might ultimately be damaging to career prospects. It is, therefore, not surprising that over the years during which it mulled over the final shape of the national alcohol policy the HPU refrained from becoming embroiled in any public debate on issues which were controversial in this sphere.

An interesting example of this distancing of itself from controversial issues is to be seen in the HPU's response to the sponsorship of the Hurling Championship by Guinness Ireland, to which reference has already been made. The voluntary codes of alcohol advertising which had evolved over many years are described in *National Alcohol Policy: Ireland,* as is their updating for broadcast media by the Minister for Arts, Culture and the Gaeltacht in 1995; the Guinness sponsorship of the Hurling Championship did not breach the 'letter of the law' of these codes, yet it could be argued that it is contrary to their general spirit and that it contravenes the WHO's *European Charter on Alcohol* which suggests that Member States:

> Implement strict controls, recognising existing limitations or bans in some countries, on direct and indirect advertising of alcoholic beverages, and ensure that no form of advertising is specifically addressed to young people, for instance, through the linking of alcohol consumption with sports.[24]

Dr Mick Loftus, a general medical practitioner and coroner for North Mayo, was a co-opted member of the Working Group which had been set up to draft the national alcohol policy; he was also a former President of the Gaelic Athletic Association (GAA) and in that capacity objected to the Guinness sponsorship of the Hurling Championship. His objections were well publicised, although ultimately futile, and he opted to absent himself from Hurling Finals – at which past Presidents of the GAA are traditionally given a place of honour – as a mark of protest. The HPU, however, made no public comment about this, nor did it play any role in fostering the growth of *Dóthain,* an organisation founded by Dr Loftus to encourage moderate drinking.

The most glaring example of the HPU's disinclination to become involved in lobbying activities – either on its own or as a network co-ordinator – is to be found, however, in relation to the public controversy which surrounded the implementation of the Road Traffic Act, 1994. This legislation reduced the permitted blood alcohol concentration (BAC) for drivers from 100mgs per 100ml of blood to 80mgs per 100ml, thereby bringing the Irish code broadly into line with other European jurisdictions.[25] The Road Traffic Act, 1994, in addition to lowering the permitted BAC for drivers, contained a number of other new measures which collectively represented a tougher approach to drink driving; these measures included:

- an automatic two-year driving ban for first conviction of driving over the new limit, as well as a fine of up to £1,000
- a requirement that all disqualified drivers should pass a driving test before having their licences returned
- power for a garda and a designated doctor to enter a hospital or a private dwelling so as to take a blood or urine specimen from a driver involved in a traffic accident
- power for the Minister for the Environment to vary the permissible alcohol level by regulation (as opposed to by legislation) and to set different limits for different classes of drivers.

In public health terms, this toughening of the drink-driving legislation obviously promised a much safer and healthier environment, given the generally accepted evidence that alcohol consumption slows reaction time and impairs drivers so as to significantly increase the risk of road traffic accidents.

The Road Traffic Act, 1994 was introduced by Mr Michael Smith, a Fianna Fáil Minister for the Environment at a time when Fianna Fáil and the Labour Party were in coalition. During the Second Stage debate on the legislation there was general support across the political spectrum in Dáil Éireann for its approach to drink driving. Speaking on behalf of Fine Gael, Deputy Avril Doyle said:

> The serious penalties for breaching the law will, I hope, bring about a climate of intolerance to drink driving, a greater awareness of the value of human life and of how much unnecessary death, suffering and expense could be avoided ... Perhaps, it would be honest if we admitted we are doing too little too late on this issue.[26]

Deputy Doyle went on to 'pay tribute to Mrs Gertie Sheils and Mothers Against Drunk Driving who, as a result of personal tragedy and suffering, have invested great energy and effort into increasing the collective consciousness of the nation of our appalling record of drink driving'.[27] (This was a reference to an Irish organisation, *Mothers Against Drunk Driving*, which like its international counterparts, had been formed by parents of children and young people killed by drunk drivers; its aim was to lobby for reform of the drink driving legislation.) It was recognised that this legislation, in the words of one Fianna Fáil backbencher, called for a 'social revolution in terms of the attitudes of Irish people to drink driving',[28] but with the exception of Deputy Austin Deasy of Fine Gael most deputies seemed to think that popular opinion had now swung in favour of such a revolution. Deputy Deasy began his contribution by making it clear that he did not condone drunken driving, but then went on to argue that the reduction in the legally permissible BAC was excessive, that it would be particularly hard on people living in rural areas and that 'We can be too puritanical at times.'[29]

The new legislation came into effect on 2 December, 1994, provoking over the subsequent two months a public debate of unprecedented ferocity, which appeared to confirm the political astuteness of Austin Deasy. Those opposed to the legislation included from the outset the various retailing bodies – the Vintners' Federation of Ireland, the Licensed Vintners' Association and the Irish Hotel Federation – and, as the campaign against the new law developed, they were joined by Dáil deputies, particularly those representing rural constituencies. Unusually, and perhaps reflecting some of its own internal organisational conflicts of this period, the Garda Representative Association (GRA) publicly opposed the new penalties; this public opposition of the GRA to the new drink-driving law drew an immediate critical response from the Garda Commissioner, who argued that the police role was one of enforcement and that the GRA should leave law-making to the elected legislators.[30]

Support for the new legislation, during this two-month period of intense public debate, came from the Irish Medical Organisation, the National

Safety Council, the Automobile Association, Mothers Against Drunk Driving, and a range of individuals – some of them, like Dr Mick Loftus, who were already seasoned campaigners and others who were less accustomed to public debate.

From a policy analysis perspective, the debate was interesting since it involved discussion not just of drink-driving issues but of the wider role played by alcohol in Irish social and cultural life. As a spectator event, this controversy was exciting and at times highly entertaining, since both sides expressed themselves forcefully on this most emotive of topics. Those opposed to the new law generally described it as draconian, suggesting that its enforcement over the Christmas period had created a reign of terror which had economically ruined the drinks trade and destroyed the social fabric and mental health of the country, and of rural areas in particular. By 23 December, for instance, Frank Fell of the Licensed Vintners' Association and Tadhg O'Sullivan of the Vintners' Federation were reporting that their members had experienced a disastrous Christmas. Frank Fell announced dramatically that 'the Christmas is finished' and that predictions that 400 jobs would be lost in the Dublin bars would have to be revised upwards 'to thousands if this continues'.[31] Describing the rural situation, Tadhg O'Sullivan pronounced it to be 'chronic at the moment' with the 'gardaí being put in a position where they are likely to lose the support of the community not through any fault of the gardaí'.[32]

While the support of the Irish Medical Organisation, the Health Research Board and a number of coroners for the new law was reported in the newspapers,[33] the tone of many independent columnists was scathing in its rejection of the tougher penalties. In the *Irish Times,* for example, Nuala O'Faoláin suggested that 'Michael Smith will be remembered, for one sole thing – for the Christmas no-one dared use the car',[34] while, in a more venomous tone, her colleague Kevin Myers lambasted the Dáil deputies who had let through this 'odious Bill' which was so culturally inappropriate to Ireland. He went on:

> We were told early this year that over 300 people had failed breath tests last Christmas. This, no doubt, would have been a splendid use of resources in the northern wastes of Sweden where news desks go on red alert and police-leave is cancelled if it is suspected that there is a driver on the roads who has recently consumed a liqueur chocolate. But in this Republic, it was a bizarre and almost immoral squandering of State resources.[35]

As a final example of this spirited debate, the Christmas *Sunday Tribune* reported that Dr Patricia Casey, 'a leading professor of psychiatry and member of the Medical Council', was opposed to the new drink-driving laws which she saw as extreme and as inimical to the mental health of men:

Professor Casey, who stresses she is totally opposed to drunk driving, points out that the 'pub culture is very important for men, particularly as their roles are challenged in modern society, often by women'.

'Where else, if not to the pub, have many men to go to relax?' she asks. 'It is often their only contact with other men on a social level and it is even more valuable to them because it is sometimes all-male ...'

Professor Casey says it would be unfortunate if the pub, 'a social setting where people meet friends and neighbours to chat about sport and politics' were to be abandoned out of fear of the new legislation.

'... Another factor worth considering', she says, is that the 'problem drinker will drink and drive anyway ...'[36]

On 24 January 1995, the two vintners' associations organised a protest march to Dáil Éireann which was estimated to have drawn a crowd of 3,000 protesters.[37] By this date, there had been a change of Government; the new Government consisting of the so-called 'Rainbow' coalition of Fine Gael, Labour, and the Democratic Left, with Fianna Fáil now consigned to opposition. The new Minister for the Environment was Mr Brendan Howlin, who had spent the previous two years as Minister for Health and who had introduced *Shaping a Healthier Future*, the health strategy document which had explicitly invoked health promotion principles. Notwithstanding this personal familiarity with health promotion – as well, presumably, as some familiarity with the work of the HPU on the drafting of a national alcohol policy – Mr Howlin agreed to an immediate review of the penalties for drink driving contained in the new legislation and, on 7 March 1995, he announced a series of amendments. The 80mg BAC was retained as the legal limit, but penalties were scaled on the basis of the degree to which BACs exceeded this limit: for example, drivers whose BAC was 81-100mgs were disqualified for just three months on a first conviction, while those whose BAC was 101-150mgs were disqualified for a year on first conviction. The requirement that disqualified drivers should have to pass a driving test before being allowed to regain their licenses was dropped for all routine disqualifications.

This softening of the penalties for drink driving just two months after the legislation came into effect was welcomed by politicians of all parties, as it was by the vintners, despite their expressions of regret that Mr Howlin had not restored the 100mg limit. The only well-publicised repudiation of the Minister's decision was that of Gertie Sheils of the Mothers Against Drunk Drivers group:

Ms Sheils said the reduction of penalties for drunken driving was 'a victory for vested interests'. She added: 'They [the publicans] gave an ultimatum to the Government to do something with the law and that is what has happened. The Government capitulated. Are we going to see every law changed to suit a vested interest group?'

'We are totally devastated by this watering down of the new Road Traffic Act which we felt was a deterrent. The penalties were the real deterrent and once you start watering down the law people lose respect for the law.[38]

The politicians, who had endured an unusually intense and bruising public debate on this topic for the months of December 1994 and January 1995, undoubtedly did not agree with this conclusion of Gertie Sheils; the view expressed by Deputy Avril Doyle – that the Road Traffic Act, 1994 was 'too little too late' – now seemed like a serious political miscalculation. In revising the penalties for drunk driving, the politicians appear to have accepted that opposition to the new legislation was widespread and enduring, rather than an ephemeral phenomenon largely created and sustained by the drinks industry.

From a health promotion perspective, the Road Traffic Act, 1994 could be seen as an example of intersectoral collaboration in which Department of the Environment legislation served an obvious public health purpose. Despite the fact that it was ostensibly engaged in formulating a national alcohol policy and therefore might be expected to welcome and publicly support this legislation, the HPU remained mute throughout this entire controversy. By remaining aloof from the debate, the HPU clarified – if clarification were necessary – its position as a traditional civil service section which opted to look back cautiously into its parent department rather than commit itself to a public role in leading and shaping the effort to retain the Road Traffic Act, 1994. Perhaps to expect otherwise was naïve: the doctrine of 'corporation sole' which has already been alluded to regards all departmental activity as ministerial activity, and it would have been difficult for civil servants in the HPU to take on a high-profile lobbying role on this issue when their minister showed no inclination to do so. Furthermore, the apparent ease and speed with which Brendan Howlin moved from his position as a health promoting Minister for Health to a Minister for the Environment who reduced the severity of penalties for drunk driving must have confirmed for civil servants that political commitment to health promotion was largely rhetorical.

One can speculate that if this debate had taken place in the United Kingdom, a major role would have been played by Alcohol Concern – precisely because Alcohol Concern is an autonomous health promotion agency rather than a central government department. Whether or not it would have made any difference to the political outcome of this episode, the major public health message that might have been articulated by an active health promotion agency concerns the common usage of the phrase 'drunken drivers' and the implied suggestion that such drivers are categorically different from ordinary responsible drivers who simply happen to have taken a few drinks. Just as the public health perspective generally suggests that the categorical distinction between *alcoholics* and *social drinkers* is illusory and that alcohol-related problems are to be found across a spectrum of drinkers, so too does it argue that risk and actual accidents are not confined to a separate category of habitual, heavy-drinking drivers. The comment of Professor Casey to the effect that the reduction of the BAC to the new limit of 80mgs would be ignored by 'problem drinkers' might have been met with the rejoinder that, since problem drinkers were in a minority in any event, the major public health benefit would accrue from the observance of the law by the vast majority of drivers whose alcohol consumption was moderate to start with. From a public health perspective, the primary aim of the drink driving law is not to punish a deviant minority of 'drunken drivers' but to deter drivers as a whole from increasing the risk of road traffic accidents.[39] However, the main point is that the HPU did not become involved in this debate and that the connection between the Road Traffic Act, 1994 and the public health perspective on alcohol was not expressed clearly and publicly throughout this entire episode.

Reorienting the health services

Finally, it is necessary to consider whether, at a time when the Department of Health was engaged in the task of formulating a national alcohol policy along health promotion lines, it made any progress in 'reorienting the health service', that is in challenging or diminishing the dominance of the alcoholism treatment ethos within the Irish health care system. This subject has already been dealt with extensively for an earlier period (1973-1988) in Chapter Three, but the issues remain essentially the same: was it possible to divert resources away from specialist alcoholism services, either towards interventions to be delivered at primary health care level or towards activities which were specifically preventive? Given the general popularity of the disease concept, the specific impact of Alcoholics Anonymous and the Irish National Council on Alcoholism, and the advent of the Minnesota Model, it would seem obvious that attempts to reorient the health services in this way were bound to be difficult.

One health promotion strategy which was particularly popular in the United Kingdom during the 1980s can be regarded, in terms of the Ottawa Charter, either as an example of reorienting health services or, alternatively, as an example of developing personal skills: the strategy in question consists of advice-giving to individual drinkers concerning the relationship between level of consumption and risk for various forms of alcohol-related problems.[40] The logic of this health promotion strategy was, of course, diametrically opposed to that inherent in the disease concept, which regarded consumption levels as unimportant in the light of its general preoccupation with vulnerability as an inherited individual factor. As it gained popularity in Britain, the trend was towards advice-giving – either through individual contact, as in the patient-GP relationship, or through media promotion – which suggested that risks could be minimised through limiting alcohol consumption to 'safe' or 'sensible' weekly levels. The consensus was that for men the safe weekly level was 21 units of alcohol, while for women it was 14 units, with a unit consisting of a British measure of spirits, a half-pint of beer or a glass of wine. The choice of these levels was somewhat arbitrary, rather than precisely scientific, but the effectiveness of the campaign was predicated upon its acceptance by the public as an authoritative, scientific statement of fact. Kendell (1987) acknowledged the arbitrary nature of the choice of safe drinking levels, adding: 'But at least we have had the wit to heed the warning Lord Melbourne gave to his cabinet about the price of corn – "It is not much matter which we say, but mind, we must all say the same".'[41]

However, despite the adoption and promotion of this preventive strategy by various royal medical colleges, the Health Education Council and Alcohol Concern, there was little evidence of its success, and in December 1995 – showing gross disregard for Lord Melbourne's warning – the British Minister for Health unilaterally raised the safe drinking limits to 28 units per week for men and 21 units per week for women. By this time, paradoxically, WHO and other authoritative thinking had come to view the concept of safe drinking levels as inaccurate and potentially harmful; strictly speaking, there is no risk-free drinking, and the publicising of these allegedly safe levels might even encourage some drinkers to increase their consumption, just as road signs may persuade motorists to drive faster when they indicate that they are driving at less than the legal speed limit. The revised public health message, while retaining the logic of the link between consumption level and risk, now consisted of the simple, but by no means unproblematic, advice that 'less is better'.

From the time of its establishment in 1988, the HPU appeared to vacillate on the subject of safe drinking level advice. In 1989, it published a 'drinking diary' and some other material which drew explicitly from British concepts and literature, but it kept all of its activities in this sphere low key and never initiated any large-scale mass media campaigns utilising this approach. By 1991, when its stock of literature was running low, the HPU was reluctant to authorise reprints, largely, it appears, on the grounds that any publicity on this topic might provoke conflict amongst members of the Working Group who were working on the national policy. Despite this, the major health strategy document *Shaping a Healthier Future* contained the following target:

To ensure that, within the next four years, 75 per cent of the population aged fifteen years and over knows and understands the recommended sensible limits for alcohol consumption. While these limits are subject to ongoing research, the present international consensus is 14 units per week for a woman and 21 units for a man.[42]

Two years later, however, when the national alcohol policy document was finally published, the HPU acknowledged that safe (or at least low risk) drinking levels were no longer being advocated and that the recommended health promotion message now consisted of the previously-mentioned dictum 'less is better'. One can regard the relative inactivity of the HPU on this issue as demonstrating shrewdness in opting not to commit itself to a health education line which quickly came to be seen as dubious; alternatively, of course, one can regard it as yet another example of civil service caution and the preoccupation with avoiding mistakes. However one chooses to interpret the HPU's activity on this front, it seems fair to conclude that health promotion of this type – which could be regarded as falling under the Ottawa Charter rubric of 'developing personal skills' – further demonstrates the difficulty and complexity of operationalising principles which in the abstract seem straightforward and non-problematic.

As already discussed in Chapter Three, the policy intent of *Planning for the Future* (1984) was to reduce admissions, lengths of stay and the general burden of alcohol problems on the Irish psychiatric hospital system. The principal means towards the realisation of this policy intent was the establishment of community-based alcohol counsellor posts within the restructured, sectorised mental health services. This policy line represented a compromise in terms of how public mental health services should handle alcohol problems, falling as it did between the extremes of simply continuing to devote large-scale hospital resources to these problems or, alternatively, refusing to allow alcohol problems to be treated at all within the psychiatric system. The rationale for this policy shift towards non-residential services was, as outlined in Chapter Three, that detoxification rarely demanded hospital admission, while evaluative research had failed to demonstrate that in-patient rehabilitation delivered outcomes superior to those of out-patient rehabilitation.

In the years succeeding the publication of *Planning for the Future* the regional health boards moved, at varying paces and with somewhat varying service structures, to create non-residential alcohol counselling services; in its *Green Paper on Mental Health* (1992) the Department of Health commented approvingly, albeit superficially, on these developments, but it never conducted any review or evaluation of these new services.

Table 6: Alcohol-related admissions as a proportion of all admissions to Irish psychiatric hospitals

Year	All admissions	Alcohol admissions (% of all admissions)
1985	29,082	7,272 (25%)
1986	29,392	7,132 (24%)
1987	27,856	6,492 (23%)
1988	28,432	6,478 (24%)
1989	27,250	6,608 (24%)
1990	27,765	6,377 (23%)
1991	27,913	6,592 (24%)
1992	27,148	6,081 (22%)
1993	27,008	5,718 (21%)
1994	26,687	5,551 (21%)
1995	26,440	5,262 (20%)

Source: Annual Activities Reports of the Medico-Social Research Board/Health Research Board

The decrease in psychiatric in-patient admissions for alcohol problems in the period 1985-1995 is illustrated in Table 6, but, as with other aspects of alcohol policy, these data are open to conflicting interpretation. Dermot Walsh continued to be in charge of the Health Research Board's mental health research programme during this period, as well as acting as Inspector of Mental Hospitals for the Department of Health. His view, stated frequently and publicly, was that the decline in alcohol-related admissions was not as speedy or as radical as he would have liked. The Report of the Inspector of Mental Hospitals for 1992, for example, included his contention that: 'Admissions for alcohol related disorders remain disturbingly high despite the Inspectorate's recommendation in recent years about the importance of providing alternative, non-residential services for this category of patient.'[43]

In most ways, however, Dermot Walsh would have to be regarded as something of a lone voice, since popular discourse and media representation of these issues still seemed to be rooted in the disease concept and, specifically, in the uncritical espousal of the value of treatment services. In 1988, for example, the *Irish Times* ran a four-part series on alcoholism which largely consisted of a rehearsal of traditional views reflecting the validity of the disease concept, and giving no real sense of how controversial or contentious this area was. The first part of this series included an uncritical presentation of American ideas about Adult Children of Alcoholics, as well as a statement from Dr Patrick

Tubridy of St John of God's Hospital, who argued – without explaining the basis for his estimate – that 'there are about 175,000 alcoholics in Ireland and for every alcoholic drinking there are 10 people who are totally miserable'.[44]

Similarly, in 1991 Dr John Cooney (while a member of the HPU's working group on a national alcohol policy) published a popular book on alcoholism in which he restated and defended the disease concept and, by implication, the value and importance of treatment. Extracts from this book were published in the *Irish Times,* again without critical comment or rebuttal. The general tenor of Cooney's advocacy of the disease concept had not changed, as may be gleaned from this quote:

> I am convinced that were it not for the disease concept of alcoholism far fewer people would have come forward for help, and might not have been encouraged to do so. Here in Ireland this concept is being threatened at the present time. If we regress to the moralistic 'sin' model of long ago, then the victims of alcohol abuse will receive the second-class treatment deemed appropriate for victims of a bad habit, self-inflicted.[45]

In early 1994, following a radio interview in which Dermot Walsh was critical of the value of or necessity for in-patient alcoholism treatment, the *Irish Medical Times* published an unsigned editorial which argued strongly against him on the basis that, *'Planning for the Future* and the *Green Paper on Mental Health* notwithstanding, the facilities available for the diagnosis and treatment of alcohol abuse are inadequate to say the least'.[46] This editorial gave rise over the next few weeks to a correspondence in the letters columns of the *Irish Medical Times* in which some of the contributors were hard-hitting in the extreme. Professor Tom Fahy of the Department of Psychiatry at University College Hospital, Galway, defended Dermot Walsh, suggesting that the editorial had been written by a private-sector psychiatrist and that psychiatrists from this background were primarily concerned to protect their commercial interests in in-patient treatment programmes. Professor Fahy also thought that a comprehensive national alcohol policy with a preventive or health promotional rationale was the best way forward, and that psychiatrists should admit that they had relatively little to contribute in this sphere.[47]

One interesting example of the ability of those who favoured in-patient treatment to lobby for the retention of structured in-patient programmes is to be found in the events which took place at St Brigid's Hospital, Ballinasloe, in early 1995. This hospital, owned and run by the Western Health Board, had set up a residential alcoholism programme in 1980 catering for about fifteen patients who typically stayed for six weeks. Three nurses from the hospital had been trained as counsellors by the Irish

National Council on Alcoholism and had worked exclusively in this service thereafter. These nurse counsellors resisted organisational pressure to transfer to community alcohol service posts during the early 1990s, and when the Health Board attempted in 1995 to close the unit (which had been housed across the road from the main hospital in a former doctors' residence) former patients of the unit mobilised and enlisted the help of local and national politicians, to successfully resist its closure. The fate of the unit was debated at a meeting of the Western Health Board and at a special meeting of Ballinasloe Urban Council, and received extensive coverage in the local press. Part of the case made by those who lobbied successfully for the retention of St Brigid's Unit was that its existence merely gave to medical card holders what VHI subscribers took for granted – in-patient rehabilitation which could never be adequately replaced by out-patient counselling services.[48]

Given this degree of contentiousness about the respective merits of in-patient and out-patient treatment programmes and the residual popularity of hospital admissions, it is perhaps not surprising that the Department of Health made no dramatic effort to reorient the health services in respect of alcoholism treatments. While, as stated above, no comprehensive evaluation of the newly established community alcohol services took place, there are some grounds for believing that rather than providing an alternative for problem drinkers who would otherwise occupy hospital beds, these services generated a new clientele. Much of the counsellors' work was with 'concerned persons', that is spouses and other relatives or associates of problem drinkers, or with problem drinkers whose difficulties were unlikely to result in hospitalisation. This is not to say, of course, that counselling with such clients is undesirable, but merely to point out that its development and scale was an unanticipated consequence of the decision to create specialist community alcohol counsellor posts. Furthermore, despite the intent to retain alcohol counsellors as an integral part of the mental health services, it was not clear that any of the health boards had succeeded in integrating community-based counselling with in-patient treatment systems.

Conclusion

The aim of this chapter was to assess the newly-established health promotion structures in terms of their performance in formulating and implementing a national alcohol policy. It was suggested from the outset that this task seemed excessively ambitious in view of the success of the disease concept in resisting the public health perspective during the period leading up to 1988. The debate surrounding the enactment of the

Intoxicating Liquor Act, 1988 once again confirmed that the policy climate had not become noticeably 'drier' or more receptive to a national alcohol policy along health promotional lines, although the Minister for Health created expectations of such a policy development through his decision to assign this task to the Advisory Council on Health Promotion and the HPU. However, the Advisory Council never functioned as the autonomous body envisaged in these early and relatively heady days of health promotion; indeed for almost all of the period considered in this chapter it never functioned at all. To some extent this is attributable to the deaths of the first two chairpersons and the political career of the third, but it also suggests that neither at Ministerial nor at civil service levels was there any real commitment to this particular structure. It is even more important to note that the Cabinet Sub-Committee on Health Promotion was little more than a fiction throughout this period, and certainly there is no evidence of political commitment at this high level to the drafting and implementation of a national alcohol policy.

The HPU remained in firm control of the formulation of the national policy document, therefore, and it has been argued here that its management of this task reflected a preoccupation with the avoidance of controversy. The organisational networks model of policy formulation, with its emphasis on negotiation and the establishment of informal alliances, simply did not fit the style of the HPU, which was after all a section of a central government department. The hollowness of the rhetoric of intersectoral collaboration was shown up particularly during the intense debate which followed the implementation of the Road Traffic Act, 1994; during this debate on alcohol consumption, driving and risk, the HPU remained silent rather than, as might have been expected, coming to the assistance of beleaguered colleagues in the Department of the Environment.

In their summary of relevant international research and its implications for alcohol policy, Edwards et al (1994) argued that:

> Alcohol problems have too often been left to the ebb and flow. It is the job of policy so far as possible to capture and control that tide in the public interest.[49]

Applying this metaphor to the period 1988-1996, the HPU must surely have seen itself as cast in the role of King Canute; the tide of alcohol consumption and related problems which it was expected to tackle or reverse seemed immune to all conventional policy responses. The use of fiscal measures to limit consumption, which is advocated in international literature, was particularly difficult in a country where alcohol consumption is price inelastic, and where, in any event, Ireland's membership of the EU does not readily allow it to increase the price of what is by European standards an already expensive commodity. Similarly, there is little political or public support for other alcohol control measures. The popularity of the disease concept and of treatment services also makes it difficult to advocate any radical reorientation of the treatment system, and there was no groundswell of popular support for such a reorientation from local community groups or regional health boards during this time.

Perhaps the main conclusion, therefore, is that the period from 1945 onwards was characterised in Ireland by an incremental drift towards an alcohol policy where the disease concept was dominant. Attempts to apply health promotion concepts, however rational such concepts appear or however sincere their advocates, had no success in terms of *realpolitik*. In Chapter Eight these issues will be considered again in relation to and in comparison with policy on illicit drugs, which forms the subject matter of Chapters Five, Six and Seven.

NOTES

1. C. Kelleher (ed.), *The Future for Health Promotion.* (Centre for Health Promotion Studies, University College Galway, 1992), p.133.
2. *Dáil Debates* (Vol. 379), Column 1992.
3. *Dáil Debates* (Vol. 379), Column 2017. It should be noted that INCA, by way of death-bed conversion, had changed its name to Irish National Council on Alcohol a few months prior to its closure.
4. *Seanad Debates* (Vol. 119), Column 1970.
5. Ibid., Column 1565.
6. *Dáil Debates* (Vol. 380), Column 1701.
7. *Dáil Debates* (Vol. 379), Column 2297.
8. M. Morgan and J. Grube, *Drinking Among Post-Primary School Pupils.* (Dublin: Economic and Social Research Institute, 1994).
9. This notice, over the name of Dr Ciarán Barry, Chairman of the Advisory Council on Health Promotion, was published in most Irish broadsheet newspapers during the first week of February, 1991.
10. Members of the Advisory Council on Health Promotion who remained on the National Alcohol Policy Working Group were: Dr John Cooney (Psychiarist); Ms Eilis Fitzpatrick (Public Health Nurse); Professor Cecily Kelleher (Professor of Health Promotion, UCG).
    Those co-opted were: Mr Shane Butler (Addiction Studies, TCD); Professor Eileen Kane (Department of Anthropology, St Patrick's College, Maynooth); Dr Mick Loftus (GP and Coroner for North Mayo); Mr Paddy Moriarty (Chairman, ESB); Mr Chris Murphy (Drug Awareness Programme, Catholic Social Services Conference, Dublin); Mr Michael Walsh (Programme Manager, Special Hospital Programme, Eastern Health Board).
    The Working Group was chaired by Mr Noel Usher, Principal Officer, Health Promotion Unit; other HPU officials who contributed were: Mr Gerry Coffey; Ms Anna-May Harkin; Ms Carmel Tobin.

Much of the following account of the formulation of the national alcohol policy is drawn from this writer's recollection of events as a member of the Working Group and from the group's business papers.

Perhaps the most notable omission from the Working Group was Dr Dermot Walsh, whose national and international reputation in the alcohol research field might have been expected to gain him an automatic place on this group.

11. The phrase 'broadly based' seems to have had a curious attraction for the HPU; it was often used in a positive sense to justify the make-up of the Advisory Council on Health Promotion, yet it was used in this instance (the first real task of the Advisory Council) to suggest that the Advisory Council was unsuited to a specific policy formulation exercise.

12. This report, *A Literature Review of Social Indicators of Alcohol Consumption in Ireland*, was compiled by Abdullahi Osman El-Tom of the Department of Anthropology, St Patrick's College, Maynooth. It was completed in April 1992.

13. Letter to Shane Butler from the Chairman of the Working Group (March 12, 1992).

14. Letter to Shane Butler from Chairman of the Working Group (February 4, 1993).

15. *Green Paper on Mental Health.* (Dublin: Stationery Office, 1992), p.26.

16. *Shaping a Healthier Future: A Strategy for Effective Healthcare in the 1990s.* (Dublin: Stationery Office, 1994), p.22.

17. *A Health Promotion Strategy: Making the Healthier Choice the Easier Choice.* (Dublin: Department of Health, 1995), p.22.

18. 'Policy on alcoholism', *Irish Medical Times,* 13 October, 1995.

19. *National Alcohol Policy – Ireland.* (Dublin: Stationery Office, 1996).

20. *Irish Times,* 20 September, 1996.

21. Ibid.

22. The statistics on Irish alcohol consumption contained in *National Alcohol Policy – Ireland* confirmed this trend; in line with the improved performance of the Irish economy, consumption which had plateaued during the 1980s begin to rise again in the 1990s.

23. *National Alcohol Policy – Ireland*, cit. sup., p.47.

24. Strategy 10 from *European Charter on Alcohol, cit. sup.*

25. The permitted BAC varies considerably from one jurisdiction to another: in the UK it is 80mg, in Germany 80mg, in France 70mg, in the Netherlands 50mg and in Sweden 20mg.

26. *Dáil Debates* (Vol. 433), Column 780.

27. *Dáil Debates* (Vol. 433), Column 782.

28. This comment was made by a Fianna Fáil deputy, Batt O'Keefe *(Dáil Debates,* (Vol. 433, Column 913).

29. *Dáil Debates* (Vol.433), Column 832.

30. 'Culligan says GRA views on drink-driving irresponsible', *Irish Times,* 23 December, 1994.

31. 'Controversy over drink-driving law intensifies', *Irish Times,* 23 December, 1994.

32. Ibid.

33. 'Doctors are fully behind drink rigour', *Irish Press,* 23 December, 1994.

34. 'Nuala O'Faoláin, 'Attitudes to drinking need fine tuning, not hammering', *Irish*

Times, 2 January, 1995.

35. Ibid.

36. 'Drink law has social risk', *Sunday Tribune,* 23/24/25 December, 1994.

37. This estimate of the size of the vintners' protest is from the *Evening Press,* 24 January, 1995.

38. Ibid.

39. For an authoritative discussion of all the policy issues involved in drink-driving legislation see H. Ross, *Confronting Drunk Driving: Social Policy for Saving Lives.* (Yale University Press, 1992).

40. Sensible drinking advice of this type was presented in a relatively popular way in: Royal College of Psychiatrists, *Alcohol: Our Favourite Drug.* (London: Tavistock, 1986).

41. R. Kendell, 'Drinking Sensibly', *British Journal of Addiction,* 82 (1987), p.1281.

42. *Shaping a Healthier Future,* cit.sup., p.49.

43. *Report of the Inspector of Mental Hospitals for the year ending 31st December 1992.* (Dublin: Stationery Office, 1995), p.3.

44. *Irish Times,* 18 April, 1988.

45. J. Cooney, *Under the Weather: Alcohol Abuse and Alcoholism – How to Cope.* (Dublin: Gill and Macmillan, 1991), p.7.

46. 'Treating alcoholism in Ireland', *Irish Medical Times,* 18 February, 1994.

47. *Irish Medical Times,* 25 February, 1994.

48. This local controversy about the closure of a residential treatment unit was covered by the *Connacht Tribune* on 7 April, 14 April and 28 April, 1995.

49. G. Edwards et al (1994), op.cit., p.212.

5

Health Policy and Illicit Drug Use in Ireland: The Early Years 1966-1979

Introduction

International drug control systems evolved and expanded throughout the twentieth century, having had their origins in the International Opium Convention of The Hague in 1912.[1] It was not, however, until the 1960s – a decade which is universally associated with increased drug use as part of a burgeoning youth culture – that health authorities in Ireland became concerned about the use of illicit psychoactive drugs, and it is the period from the mid-1960s to the mid-1990s which will be looked at in this and in the next two chapters.

Despite the existence of a high degree of support internationally for drug control systems, amounting to a consensus for all practical purposes, interesting and important policy differences emerged in this sphere between Britain and the USA during the first half of the twentieth century. In the USA, the Harrison Act, 1914, or to be precise the interpretation of this legislation by the Supreme Court, effectively gave dominance to the criminal justice system in terms of the societal management of illicit drug use. American ideological commitment to drug prohibition was strictly and consistently adhered to, with doctors being forbidden to prescribe maintenance doses for patients who could not or would not remain drug free. In Britain, on the other hand, the Rolleston Committee of 1926 established the right of medical practitoners to prescribe psychoactive drugs on a maintenance basis, where detoxification had not led to a drug-free life and where indefinite maintenance prescribing offered the prospect of social stability and a healthier lifestyle.[2]

By the time that Irish health policy makers began to address this issue, some degree of convergence had begun to emerge between these two therapeutic systems. During the 1960s, British policy makers became less convinced of the wisdom of medicalising addiction and leaving its management largely to the discretion of individual doctors, and, following the second report of the Brain Committee in 1965, prescribing rights of general medical practitioners were restricted and a specialist 'clinic' system was inaugurated. The American experience at this time was that its policy of giving total 'ownership' of drug problems to the criminal justice sector was also unsatisfactory. During the 1960s, largely through the collaborative work of Vincent Dole, a metabolic disease specialist, and Marie Nyswander, a psychiatrist, at the Rockefeller Institute in New York, American policy and practice changed, albeit partially and grudgingly, to allow for the creation of maintenance programmes for opiate addicts. This Dole and Nyswander system of maintenance, which is now practised more or less universally, involves the use of methadone, a synthetic opiate, rather than heroin; methadone is a long-acting drug which provides its users with relief from withdrawal symptoms through a single daily dose and which, if prescribed at a sufficiently high dosage, may reduce the incentive for simultaneous use of street heroin by virtue of its so-called 'blockade' effect.

By the time, therefore, that Irish policy makers came to address drug issues in the mid-1960s, it was already clear from the international experience that the provision of treatment services within the overall framework of drug prohibition was a complex and contentious matter. The primary aim of eliminating the supply of drugs, even when supported by tough criminal justice sanctions, had not been achieved and, arguably, was never going to be achieved. There was, it appeared, a universal demand for mind-altering drugs, a demand that was resistant to both supply reduction and demand reduction strategies. Equally importantly perhaps, there was no medical technology which could effectively stop people using drugs if that was their choice, and treatment policy was caught between insisting that detoxification and rehabilitation – aimed at achieving a drug-free status – should be the sole activity of the health care system or accepting that some form of harm minimisation or harm reduction interventions – such as methadone maintenance for opiate dependence – was also a legitimate option.

The Working Party on Drug Abuse, 1968-1971

In studying Irish policy on illicit drugs from the 1960s onwards, it is convenient to start by considering the *Working Party on Drug Abuse,* the first official committee to examine drug problems in Ireland and to make recommendations as to future policy. The background to the establishment of this Working Party will be discussed in detail later in this section, but for the moment it is sufficient to note that it was set up by the Minister for Health, Seán Flanagan, in December 1968 with the following terms of reference:

To examine the extent of drug abuse in Ireland at present; to advise the Minister
on the steps which might be taken to deal with the problem, including measures
to discourage young persons from starting the use of drugs (e.g. publicity,
education, example, etc.); to advise on the action to be taken to assist in the
rehabilitation of persons who have acquired the drug habit.[3]

The 1966 *Report of the Commission of Inquiry on Mental Illness* had
touched briefly on the subject of drug use and addiction, concluding that
while there was no evidence of a drug scene in Ireland at this time: 'The
Commission considers that drug addiction could reach serious proportions
in this country unless a constant effort is maintained to prevent the abuse
of habit-forming drugs'.[4] The Department of Health did not begin any
formal monitoring of illicit drug use or related problems in the wake of this
recommendation, nor did it initiate any other policy development in this
area; but, as will now be discussed, it set up the Working Party on Drug
Abuse some two years later – somewhat reluctantly it would appear – as a
result of ongoing lobbying and media coverage of the drugs issue.[5]

In explaining the events leading up to the establishment of the Working
Party on Drug Abuse by the Minister for Health, the role played by the
Garda Síochána and, in particular, the networking skills of Sergeant Denis
Mullins of the Garda Drug Squad cannot be over-emphasised. The
'Special Branch' was the name popularly given in the 1960s to that section
of the Garda Síochána which had responsibility for political and
paramilitary crime and which also liaised with international policing
organisations. Denis Mullins, who was a detective sergeant in the Special
Branch, had become convinced from the mid-1960s that illicit drug use in
the Dublin area was becoming more common and causing more problems,
although at this time there was no official acceptance of this point of view.
While some drugs were being imported from abroad either by users
themselves or by small-time drug dealers, it appeared to Mullins that the
main source of supply for the emerging drug scene in Dublin came from
robberies of chemist shops and Dublin Health Authority dispensaries. His
first successful venture into drug policy was to persuade his own
authorities, in 1967, to set up a small specialist unit within the Garda
Síochána, and he himself headed up this 'Drug Squad' despite his
relatively low rank. Belying all stereotypes of police officers as cautious,
conservative and incapable of communication except through their own
internal hierarchy, Denis Mullins made contacts across a range of
interested individuals and groups who could help him in lobbying for
policy development in the drugs field. These contacts were with a variety
of people – psychiatrists, pharmacists, social workers, teachers, priests and
journalists – and he created a reputation for being caring and
compassionate towards drug users, rather than being solely committed to

law enforcement and to securing convictions. Dr Noel Browne, for instance, who was part of the Denis Mullins network, commented in Dáil Éireann at the committee stage of the Health Bill, 1969 that the Garda Síochána were 'wonderfully understanding in their approach to and handling of this problem'.[6]

It is interesting to compare the work of Denis Mullins on this issue with that of Mr Christy O'Connor of the College of Pharmacy, who also became a lobbyist for drug policy development. Christy O'Connor was drawn into the Mullins network initially to do laboratory analysis of seized drugs and to provide expert testimony in court, but went on to develop a much wider interest in drug policy. Recalling the efforts which he made to have drug problems recognised by the authorities, he told a journalist subsequently:

> They kept dismissing the reports that drug abuse was a growing problem. They always referred to it as being a small problem in comparison to the enormous alcohol problem. They seemed to want to damp down anxiety about it. But not only were the government and courts lacking in knowledge about the problems of drug abuse but doctors and pharmacists were also oblivious to the problems.
>
> I found in my work on drug abuse that two significant factors in the spread of drug abuse was [sic] the overprescribing of dangerous drugs by doctors and the almost non-existent supervision of drug supplies kept in chemist shops and dispensaries. I could see quite clearly in my work in court that they knew virtually nothing about drug abuse and cared less; that the authorities hoped that by ignoring the urgency of the problem it would go away.[7]

Although he was influential, particularly in relation to the introduction of new regulations governing amphetamines and barbiturates and the holding of drugs in chemist shops and dispensaries, Christy O'Connor did not appear to have the same networking skills as Denis Mullins, who seemed to be uniquely capable of saying difficult and challenging things without creating antagonism. Towards the end of 1968, when a critical mass of popular opinion for the review of drug policy had been achieved through lobbying and the use of the media, the Minister for Health conceded and set up the Working Party. Denis Mullins was appointed to this committee and, perhaps because the Garda Síochána were somewhat puzzled that such a junior officer would be appointed to an intersectoral governmental committee, so too was an Inspector from the Special Branch. Christy O'Connor of the College of Pharmacy was not, however, appointed to the committee.

The Working Party was based within and serviced from the Department of Health, and it is worth noting that within the Department of Health responsibility for drug issues was allocated to the Food and Drugs Section (subsequently renamed the Public Health Division) rather than to the Mental Health Section. The relevance of this allocation is that it signified that drug control systems (supply reduction) were considered more important than treatment systems (demand reduction).[8] Nonetheless, in his address to the first meeting of the Working Party, the Minister for Health pointed out that while the Government was considering legislative action to strengthen its drug control systems, it did not see criminal justice sanctions as the primary or most useful way to tackle drug problems. In addition to emphasising the importance of educating young people about the risks involved in drug use, the Minister suggested that those who developed a dependency on drugs were 'more to be pitied than punished, and should be regarded as sick people in need of medical care to be treated with sympathy and understanding and to be helped in every way possible to overcome their dependency on drugs'.[9] In short, the Ministerial view as the Working Party began its work was that Irish drug policy should combine treatment and rehabilitation activities with control measures.

Before discussing the conclusions and recommendations of the Working Party, it is important to comment briefly on what it did *not* do. The committee accepted, apparently without question, the assumptions implicit in the phrase 'drug abuse' and in the terms of reference given to it, and did not indulge itself in any philosophical or sociological scrutiny of this concept or of the apparent inevitability of prohibitionist policies. It is understandable that the Working Party should have opted to ignore fundamental debate of this kind, since to do otherwise would have made it virtually impossible to accomplish the commonsense, administrative tasks expected of it. The Working Party was aware of and referred to the 'Wooton' Report 1968, a British committee report on cannabis which had been chaired by the social scientist Baroness Barbara Wooton. It is reasonable to assume that the Working Party was also aware of the opprobrium heaped upon Wooton because of her relatively moderate proposals to reduce the penalties for cannabis convictions; these aggresssive attacks on Wooton were not just a feature of the tabloid and more conservative broadsheet newspapers in Britain, but also involved the Home Secretary of the day, James Callaghan.[10] The Irish policy climate at this time would have probably been equally, if not more, hostile to even mildly liberal proposals on drug use, and the terms of reference of the Working Party clearly pointed it in the rather conventional direction which the Minister for Health and his department wished it to go. There were, however, areas of discussion – such as the question of drug education, which will be considered later in this chapter – where critical debate could not be avoided. Finally, it is worth noting that members of the Working Party were not lacking a sense of either humour or irony; three different members of the committee told this writer that, as a team-building exercise, they had enjoyed a memorable drinks party during the early period of their deliberations, and also that the meal to mark the completion and signing of the final report became rather bibulous – with the conviction that drug abuse in Ireland had been dealt a serious blow strengthening in direct relation to the amount of alcohol consumed!

The Working Party held its first meeting in January 1969, submitted an interim report in September of that year, and completed its final report in February 1971. Viewed from a health promotional perspective, the membership of the committee was impressive, with representation from various medical specialties, pharmacy, social services, education, the criminal justice system and third-level students. The choice of Dr Karl Mullen, a well-known obstetrician and gynaecologist, as chairman of the committee was unusual, given that he had no experience of drug problems and their treatment, and it might have been expected that a psychiatrist would take on this role because of the tradition of treating addictions within the mental health system. Dr Mullen himself suggested that he had been selected for this task because of his association with sport – he had played on the Irish rugby team which had won two Triple Crowns and this might have been seen as making him an appropriate role model for young people.[11] A number of members of the committee have suggested, rather more cynically, that the choice of chairman was influenced by those civil servants who were unconvinced of the necessity of the Working Party in the first instance and who were anxious to avoid having a psychiatrist – who might use the high-profile nature of the exercise to build a personal career or empire in drugs – in this position.

The recommendations of the Working Party were largely predictable given its terms of reference; but they were, even from the perspective of more than thirty years later, well argued and clearly presented. The recommendations were balanced evenly between treatment and prevention. The whole question of treatment and rehabilitation will be dealt with in more detail later in this chapter, but it should be pointed out here that the Department of Health had effectively pre-empted the Working Party on this issue by setting up treatment services in the Dublin area during the period of the Working Party's deliberations. Recommendations for prevention included both proposals for new legislative control measures, to be backed up by tough penalties, and proposals for education and publicity aimed primarily at young people with a view to dissuading them from using drugs. The recommendations for new statutory controls were moderate and carefully considered. It was specifically argued that increased police powers should lead to 'no undue interference with the freedom of the individual';[12] that a distinction should be made between 'simple' possession and possession for the purpose of sale or supply to others; that penalties should be scaled on the basis of the kind of drug involved, and that cannabis offences should be treated in a somewhat more lenient manner. The report of the Working Party also contained the first published statistics on the prevalence of drug abuse in Dublin at this time, drawing its data mainly from Garda sources since healthcare and other data were not routinely available at this time. At the time of the Interim Report, in September 1969, there were approximately 350 persons known to the Gardaí as drug abusers in Dublin; by December 1970 this figure had grown to 940, and it was believed that this was a real increase rather than merely a reflection of increased Garda activity. The most commonly abused drugs at this time were cannabis and LSD; neither heroin nor any of the synthetic opiates were in common use and there was no evidence of large-scale commercial drug dealing.[13]

It should be pointed out in concluding this account of the Working Party on Drug Abuse that the committee viewed its brief in terms which clearly and explicitly reflected what would later come to be known as an intersectoral health promotion perspective. This perspective is expressed most succinctly in Chapter X, a short chapter towards the end of the report in which the committee states:

> We were asked by the Minister for Health to examine the problem of drug abuse but it will be clear from the wide field covered by our recommendations that the problem is far more than a 'health' matter. Thus responsibility for dealing with the problem and for implementing the various measures referred to in our report rests with a number of Government Departments, other public bodies and interested groups ... the Department of Health is essentially concerned with problems relating to treatment and epidemiological aspects of drug abuse as well as with certain aspects of the statutory controls over the availability and distribution of drugs, the Department of Justice has direct responsibility for the enforcement of these controls and for the criminal law ... The Department of Education is vitally concerned in the matters contained in our Chapter on Education and Publicity ... The Revenue Commissioners and the Department of Posts and Telegraphs have responsibilities in relation to the smuggling of drugs ...[14]

The Working Party went on, therefore, to recommend that there should be close and continuing liaison on drug issues between all Government departments, and also that a permanent advisory body on drugs, with a membership broadly similar to that of the Working Party, should be established to monitor what promised to be a changing drug scene.

What was intended to be a permanent advisory body, described as the Inter-Departmental Committee on Drug Abuse, was in fact established in 1972 in line with this latter recommendation; it was, however, a relatively informal body, serviced by the Department of Health but with no statutory basis. From a health promotion perspective, the key question to ask about this committee concerns the enthusiasm and energy which the Department of Health displayed in co-ordinating this drugs network. The Working Party had been set up by ministerial decree, following the publicity which had been largely the product of the Denis Mullins network; the Department of Health had shown no evidence of urgency or conviction concerning the need for policy development in the drugs field and – as was shown in the earlier chapters of this book on the topic of alcohol-related problems – neither did it find the networking role comfortable or congruent with its own internal organisational culture. On the whole, the answer to this key question is that the Department of Health demonstrated little commitment to managing the network of individuals and institutions represented on the Inter-Departmental Committee on Drug Abuse; however, since this was only to become evident in the early 1980s its discussion and consideration will be kept for Chapter Six.

Education and prevention

The idea of using education about drugs as a means of problem prevention was, as described above, amongst the topics included in the terms of reference of the Working Party on Drug Abuse. Attitudes towards drug education were at this time simplistic in the extreme, as exemplified in the comments of the Minister for Health during his opening address to the Working Party, when he suggested that:

> [M]any of the people taking drugs are young persons with no evil intent, taking them occasionally 'for kicks' or to be 'with it' who would, I should think, have nothing to do with drugs if they were properly advised and informed of the harmful consequences of continuing to take them.[15]

However, once it began its study of preventive drug education the Working Party quickly discovered how complex and contentious this subject was. Initially, the assumption was that factual drug education could function as a form of cognitive immunisation more or less as the Minister had suggested. It was envisaged that outside experts would address captive audiences of young people, most commonly in schools, to explain the risks inherent in drug use and to advise them to reject illicit drugs should they be offered them, and it was presumed that information and admonition of this kind would be sufficient to deter most young people from experimenting with drugs. This approach to drug education was, of course, similar to that pursued by the Irish National Council on Alcoholism since its inception in 1966: in the case of alcoholism education the outside experts tended to be either treatment specialists or recovering alcoholics.

The Working Party also contemplated using a broadly similar philosophy for the proposed publicity campaign aimed at the general public, where it was intended to use the mass media for communicating an anti-drugs message.

Underlying these proposals was an implicit belief that drug abuse was a self-evident, discrete pathological entity which could be defined in objective scientific terms. Accordingly, it was assumed that scientists could provide an authoritative, value-free legitimation of drug control systems, and that this legitimation could then be used to underpin all drug education programmes. Beliefs of this kind did not survive for long, however, once the Working Party immersed itself in the details of drug education. It became apparent that there was no scientific consensus on either what constituted 'drug abuse' or the effectiveness of the simple information-giving approach to drug education originally envisaged. A study by a British psychologist (Wiener, 1970) which was consulted by the Working Party raised a number of these difficulties; one concerned cannabis specifically and suggested that giving honest information to school-children about this drug was likely to have the opposite effect to that desired, while another was that a universalist implementation of drug education programmes was likely to arouse interest in large numbers of children who had previously not considered using drugs.[16]

Draft proposals on drug education, based on simple information-giving, were circulated by the Working Party to a number of psychologists and youth workers, but generally the response from these parties was critical. For example, E.F. O'Doherty, who was Professor of Psychology at University College Dublin, while aware that he was 'being negative, but I hope not unhelpful', made a number of fundamental criticisms of the draft document on drug education which he had been sent. He argued that: '"Straightforward information-giving" is likely to arouse experimental approach in the young rather than deter. There is considerable evidence that this is so'. On the question of mass media campaigns, he was equally critical of what was proposed:

> With regard to the content of page 4: 'Publicity and adult education', it seems to me that instead of such massive use of communications media, public agencies etc., I would strongly suggest a cool playing down of the problem. I strongly believe, and I think it could be shown that the very devices suggested on this page are calculated to create problems rather than solve them.[17]

Another critical response came from the Rev. Patrick McDermott, who was Secretary of the Youth Welfare Section of the Catholic Social Welfare Bureau; he questioned the logical consistency of trying to persuade young people on moral and health grounds not to use drugs when the use of alcohol and nicotine did not seem so radically different. 'Why is alcohol in moderation socially acceptable but marjuana *[sic]* in moderation not?'[18]

What was by far the most radical critique of the draft proposals on education came, however, from two clinical psychologists in the Dublin Health Authority, Ingo Fischer and Brian Glanville. They wrote a lengthy and thoughtful response to the document they had been sent, in which they rejected the validity of the individualism which was implicit in all of the Working Party's proposals for preventive drug education. The concept of individualism in this context refers to the ideological presumption, which was common to much of health education and still has its adherents, that the health status of an individual can be viewed solely as the product of that individual's behavioural choices or lifestyle, with little or no significance being attached to social circumstances or environmental factors. Naidoo (1986), in a later theoretical critique of individualism in health education, argued succinctly that 'Three major criticisms can be levelled against individualistic health education: first, it denies that health is a social product; second, it assumes free choice exists; third, it is not effective within its own terms of reference'.[19] Fischer and Glanville argued along similar lines in 1970, when they suggested that the focus on individual decision-making being recommended by the Working Party was seriously flawed since it ignored the social circumstances which they predicted would constitute 'the major growth area for drug addicts'.[20] If the individualistic approach to drug education is equivalent to what the Ottawa Charter refers to as the task of *Developing Personal Skills,* then the broader and more politically radical recommendations of Fisher and Glanville could be categorised, in terms of the Ottawa Charter, as *Creating Supportive Environments* and/or *Strengthening Community Action.*

In brief, Fischer and Glanville predicted that the growth of serious drug problems in Dublin would be a feature of deprived neighbourhoods and would correlate with delinquency and a host of other social problems, rather than being primarily a phenomenon which would be randomly spread and largely explicable in terms of individual psychopathology. Their prediction concerning this new group of problem drug users in Dublin read, in part, as follows:

> Typically, a member of this group is likely to come for *[sic]* a Corporation Housing Estate and to have little parental control and harmony in his home, to be part of a school system which is inadequate in many respects ... the area is likely to have poor recreational facilities and the child is likely to suffer from overcrowding in his environment ...[21]

This prediction, as will be seen in Chapter Six, was to prove remarkably accurate, but the Working Party balked at endorsing (or even discussing) preventive measures which, in the words of Fischer and Glanville, demanded 'a fairly drastic re-organisation of the social structure of the municipal housing estates' and 'a redesign of both the physical and psychological environment.'[22]

The Working Party was obviously thrown by the unexpected complexity of the drug prevention debate, and appears to have vacillated between recommending that Ireland should have no drug education programmes at all and recommending forms of drug education which at least seemed to do no harm. This ambivalence is nicely illustrated in the minutes of the committee for 23 June, 1970:

> Copies of the draft report prepared by the sub-committee [Education and Publicity] had been circulated. The report in general was agreed to but it was felt that the first section of the report should be re-drafted so as to avoid the impression of an apparent contradiction as between the introductory portion which stressed that there should be no educational programme and the later section which recommended the kind of programme which should be implemented. It was felt that the introduction should omit the references to opposing view points.[23]

Ultimately, the brief chapter on drug education (Chapter VII) which appeared in the Committee's final report was a compromise. It pointed out the complexities and what appeared, at least on occasion, to be the counterproductive aspects of drug education; but it also recommended drug education for those already known to be abusing drugs or deemed to be particularly at risk. The committee's unease with this aspect of its brief is reflected explicitly in its recommendation that another committee should be established:

> A group representing the Departments of Health and Education, the schools, the university departments, and professional bodies concerned should investigate the general question of communicating information on drugs to young persons, should provide guidance for school authorities and indicate areas where research is needed. This group should include specialists who advise on medical, psychological and social aspects.[24]

The result of this recommendation was the appointment of the *Committee on Drug Education* by Erskine Childers, Minister for Health, in October 1972 under the chairmanship of Bunny Carr, a broadcaster and communications consultant. The terms of reference of this new committee were precisely those contained in the above recommendation of the Working Party, and its membership consisted of fourteen people from varied backgrounds.

The Committee on Drug Education submitted a brief interim report to the Minister for Health in February 1973, the most notable aspect of which was the suggestion that there should be a moratorium 'on all lectures and film shows on drug abuse in schools until such time as the Committee is in a position to give guidelines in the matter to school authorities.'[25] The reason for this suggested moratorium was the evidence available to the committee that drug education was becoming increasingly popular, particularly in secondary schools, but that much of this education was of a type which was likely to do no good – it tended to consist of one-off teaching sessions, usually delivered by outside speakers, and its content was sensational and exaggerated. In 1972, yet another committee – this one appointed by the Irish Council of Churches/Roman Catholic Joint Group on the Role of the Churches in Irish Society – had looked at drug issues in Ireland and, on the subject of education, had reached similar conclusions, referring not merely to exaggerated denunciations of drugs and drug use but also to: 'another hazard [which] comes from elevating drugs to a position of supreme importance by arranging talks from "star turns", particularly ex-addicts'.[26]

This latter opinion of the inter-churches group, particularly in conjunction with the proposed moratorium on schools talks, highlights the conflict between attempts to conduct rational – or what would latterly be called 'evidence-based' – drug education programmes in schools and the more popular approach to such activity. Research evidence, by and large, suggested that drug education should be low-key, conducted by teachers and aimed at developing life-skills, if it were to have a positive outcome or at least if it were to avoid being counter-productive. On the other hand, the prohibitionist nature of public policy on drugs, the harshness of the criminal justice sanctions involved and the sensationalist style of popular cultural representations of drugs all conspired to create and sustain the image of illicit drugs as being unspeakably evil. It was understandable, therefore, that school children, their parents, school management committees and perhaps the public generally should expect drug education to reflect this unambiguous and exciting truth. Teachers whose competence to teach academic subjects was unquestioned seemed to lack the credibility and verve expected of drug educators, and there was considerable demand for outside 'experts' to come into schools and tell it like it really was. This was not just an Irish phenomenon, as will be clear from the following remarks of Halleck (1970), one of the early American critics of drug education:

> Too often the program consists of one or more meetings at which a local physician, a law enforcement officer and perhaps a former addict will endlessly catalogue the horrible outcome of drug usage. The physician will exaggerate the degree to which drugs can produce bodily damage. The law enforcement officer

will gravely talk about the increasing flow of drugs into the community and will throw in a few anecdotes about young people he has seen ruined by drugs. Sometimes he will even bring in displays of confiscated drugs to show his presumably horrified audience. The former addict, who is usually the star performer, will recount his sordid experiences as a drug user and will glowingly report the salutary effects of his reformation. It is an interesting show which has much of the glamour of an old-fashioned revival meeting.[27]

In its final report, which was presented to the Minister for Health in April 1974, the Committee on Drug Education recommended that school children *should* be given education on drug use and drug problems. The committee, like the Working Party which had preceded it, favoured an individualistic model and made no reference to structural factors which might predispose some young people to having far more negative drug experiences than others. Within the confines of this individualistic approach, however, the committee resisted the pressure to succumb to the populist and propagandistic style of drug education discussed above; it recommended that drug education should not be delivered in isolation but as part of a broader health education curriculum and also that, as a rule, it should be carried out by ordinary teachers rather than outside experts. The style and content of school drug programmes favoured by the committee was also radically different from what was popularly expected; it was recommended of school programmes that:

They should avoid becoming a mere set of rules and, more especially, a set of prohibitions. Obviously such programmes would include inter-personal relationships, personal responsibility, dignity of the individual and maturity. Within this broad context, it is felt that direct drug education could be usefully given.[28]

This style of non-directive education, more akin to counselling than to traditional didactic practice, was a far cry from the 'old-fashioned revival meetings' referred to by Halleck, but it remained to be seen whether it would be implemented or what the ramifications of this broad approach to drug education might be in Ireland. The committee noted that statutory responsibility for health education lay with the health boards under Section 71 of the Health Act, 1970, but that there was little evidence of such education being carried out in Irish schools.[29] To encourage and support the development of health education generally, the committee recommended that a national health education authority should be set up under the Health (Corporate Bodies) Act, 1961. The Minister for Health, Brendan Corish, (by this time Fianna Fáil had been replaced by a Coalition Government of Fine Gael and Labour) accepted this recommendation immediately and in October 1974 announced the establishment of a *Health Education Bureau* (HEB).

Treatment and rehabilitation

It is clear from a study of this early period of Irish drug policy development that, rhetorically at least, nobody disputed the value or desirability of setting up treatment and rehabilitation services for dependent or other problem drug users. The comments of the Minister for Health to the Working Party on Drug Abuse, to the effect that people who were dependent on drugs were deserving of medical care, have already been cited, and indeed the Working Party devoted two chapters of its final report to this topic. These two chapters cannot be considered as being of any real policy importance, however, because in 1969 – two years before the Working Party reported – the Department of Health had itself taken steps to set up a drug treatment system which was to remain in place, virtually unchanged, for the next twenty years. The motivation behind this pre-empting of the Working Party may well have been that the Department of Health was convinced of the necessity to take a speedy initiative on this issue, rather than await the recommendations of a committee which was moving at the relaxed pace characteristic of official committees. Equally, of course, it may have been that the Department of Health felt that it had been wrong-footed by the effective lobbying of Denis Mullins and his associates and took this opportunity to set up services as *it* saw fit, rather than leave this matter to the Working Party.

In any event, the Working Party was presented with a *fait accompli* in the matter of treatment services, and had little option but to endorse this departmental initiative, which it did in its interim report of November 1969 as well as in its final report. It is important, therefore, to examine in detail this creation of the Jervis Street Hospital drug treatment service, which was carried out without public debate or scrutiny but which was to have such lasting effects.[30]

On 2 May, 1969, a meeting took place between representatives of the Department of Health, the Dublin Health Authority and Jervis Street Hospital (a voluntary, city-centre hospital which closed in the mid-1980s). Subsequent to this meeting, Dr Joseph Woodcock, Honorary Secretary of Jervis Street Hospital Medical Board, Dr John Ryan, Consultant Psychiatrist at Jervis Street, and Dr R.D. Stevenson, Consultant Psychiatrist at St Brendan's Hospital – a Dublin Health Authority psychiatric hospital – visited a number of British drug dependency units and drew up a plan for the creation of treatment services for drug users in Dublin. Essentially, it was decided to set up an out-patient clinic for drug addicts at Jervis Street Hospital while simultaneously creating an in-patient unit for treatment and rehabilitation at St Brendan's Hospital. The thinking of these three doctors on this topic may be readily explained in the context of the new 'clinic' system which was now being established in Britain as a result of the Second Brain Committee. As previously mentioned, British drug policy was changing at this time from the liberal Rolleston system to the more controlling style of the Second Brain Committee, and it was this less liberal set of ideas and institutions which now recommended itself to the visiting Dublin doctors. In short, the model of drug treatment and rehabilitation which was now favoured in Britain and which was being imported into Ireland was one which emphasised the value of centralised and specialist services, with a minimal role for primary health care or localised service provision. It is probably as important to consider the policy process which led to the creation of the Dublin drug treatment system as it is to examine its content. The British had just changed from a policy which had been in place for forty years, following a study of the old system and a review of possible alternatives by a public committee. The Department of Health in Ireland, on the other hand, with no history of drug treatment provision prior to this, had accepted this recent revision of British policy more or less axiomatically, and had set up services along these lines without any public discussion or critical debate on this subject; in doing so it had pre-empted any views which the Working Party on Drug Abuse – its own expert group – might have had on this important topic.

The selection of Jervis Street Hospital as the site for the out-patient drug treatment centre was explained in the unpublished planning document in terms of the experience of the London clinics which the three Dublin doctors had visited. It was suggested that general hospitals were more acceptable for the provision of out-patient services to addicts and their families than psychiatric hospitals, and it was also seen as helpful that they offered emergency medical care and laboratory facilities for screening blood and urine – facilities usually not available in psychiatric hospitals. Jervis Street Hospital was seen to satisfy all of these criteria, and it was also seen as advantageous that it had an existing Poisons Information Centre and a city-centre location.

The thinking behind the location of the in-patient treatment centre was briefly presented as follows:

> We feel that in-patient facilities are best suited in a psychiatric hospital where they will have available to them the background system and expertise of residential psychiatric nursing and other ancillary facilities. St Brendan's Hospital appears to be the most suitable hospital to provide the in-patient service.[31]

While there was again only the briefest of discussions of treatment policy – and no attempt at setting the recent British policy changes within the context of the previous regime – it was conceded that, for the small number of opiate dependent persons for whom it appeared necessary, methadone maintenance should be available in Jervis Street. Given the nature of Irish drug treatment services as they were to evolve after 1969, there was also the rather provocative and disingenuous recommendation that 'The policy of Treatment Centres in Ireland should create conditions here which are less attractive than those in Great Britain and thus inhibit any possibility of a migration towards this country'.[32]

This latter comment gives some indication of the negative view of drug addicts contained in this planning document, a view which contrasts sharply with the conventional wisdom on alcoholism and alcoholics described in earlier chapters. If alcoholics were seen as innocent victims of a baffling disease, if not indeed as rather more noble and more sensitive than those who appeared to be able to drink with impunity, attitudes towards those dependent on illicit drugs were much less benign. Implicit in this document was the notion that drug addicts were behaviourally difficult and devious patients who would have to be monitored closely and kept at some remove from generic services and facilities. While it was argued on page one of the document that Jervis Street Hospital, as a general hospital, would be attractive to addicts, page three contained the following statement:

> We think that such a Clinic situated at Jervis Street Hospital should be separated from the other out-patient facilities and that the individuals attending should be isolated from the general hospital. This will be necessary because of the tendency of addicts to seek drugs and to interfere with the management of ordinary patients.[33]

The document later suggested that 'The services of a porter would also be a necessity on account of the character of the patients attending'.[34] While it did not say what precisely this character was, the implication seemed stereotypically negative.

The importance of this planning process which took place outside the ambit of the Working Party on Drug Abuse – *inter alia* formally charged with the task of planning rehabilitation services – became even greater in the light of the decision not to confine the functions of the Jervis Street Centre to clinical matters. It was recommended that it should 'also serve as an advisory centre for parents, individuals concerned with social problems associated with addiction, consultation with the legal authorities, advice to schools and [that] in general it should take a leading role in the organisation of a system of prevention of spread of addiction'.[35] This was a very ambitious agenda for a small centre which was to be staffed quite modestly[36] and which was clearly going to be peripheral to the activities of

Jervis Street Hospital as a whole. When the centre opened in late 1969 it was based in a caravan in the hospital courtyard, where it remained for more than a year before moving to a pre-fabricated building alongside the hospital's out-patient department. In 1971 a full-time medical director, Dr Michael Kelly (a consultant psychiatrist), was appointed and at about this time the Jervis Street Centre designated itself as the *National Drug Advisory and Treatment Centre.* The role of this unit in the period following 1979, when there was a major increase in heroin use in Dublin, will be explored further in Chapter Six.

It is instructive, however, to consider the fate of the in-patient addiction unit at St Brendan's Hospital which was intended to complement the Jervis Street service. In December 1969, the Minister for Health, Erskine Childers, officially opened this unit which was known as St Dymphna's. Although it had been specifically established as a treatment centre for drug-related problems, its medical director, Dr Stevenson, opted from the start to make its facilities available to both alcoholics and drug addicts. This was an unusual decision, since the psychiatric services generally at this time were dealing with increasing numbers of alcoholics while showing little or no interest in drug addiction. Within a year of its opening, however, the Eastern Health Board (as the Dublin Health Authority had now become) decided that St Dymphna's would only be used for the treatment of alcoholics, and its effective closure as a drug treatment centre left Jervis Street with a monopoly in this field. It is a measure of the blandness of the Working Party's coverage of treatment issues that it merely reported that: 'A special unit for the treatment of drug abusers and alcoholics was subsequently established at St Brendan's Hospital, Dublin, but this joint arrangement did not prove successful and the operation was discontinued for drug cases.'[37]

It seems unusual that a new unit which had been resourced and opened specifically for the treatment of drug addicts should abandon its task in such a peremptory way, and it seems even more unusual that neither the Department of Health nor the Eastern Health Board thought it necessary to question why this happened. In fact, the decision to stop treating drug addicts in St Dymphna's was the result of the difficulties which its staff experienced in running the unit as a joint response to alcohol and drug problems.[38] The drug addicts and alcoholics appeared to feel a great mutual antipathy towards one another and the resulting conflict militated against the creation of a therapeutic milieu. In these circumstances, it might reasonably be expected that the staff of St Dymphna's and the administrators of the Eastern Health Board would opt to exclude the alcoholics and continue to offer a service to drug addicts; instead, because alcoholics were more numerous and because they were more easily managed and less challenging of the treatment system, the decision was that the service to drug addicts should be discontinued. At one level, this abandonment of the St Dymphna's service to drug addicts within a year of its establishment appears to be explicable in terms of poor planning and inadequate staff training – rather than being the inevitable result of natural incompatibilities between two groups of patients. Drug addicts were generally younger than alcoholics and much less prepared to defer to the authority of the psychiatric system, but the successful management of alcoholics and drug addicts within a single facility is, of course, possible once clear treatment philosophies and definite institutional structures are in place. At a more fundamental level, however, the closure of St Dymphna's as a drug treatment facility signalled what was to become a more enduring feature of the Irish health service response to addicts and problem drug users, namely the tendency of mainstream health service systems and professionals to distance themselves from illicit drug users, whatever the rhetoric about creating a caring approach.

Two further services for drug addicts were established within the Eastern Health Board's psychiatric system, one a small, closed residential unit at the Central Mental Hospital in Dundrum and the other a day centre at Usher's Island, but a review of their activities suggests the same difficulty and discomfort in adapting to the needs of this new client population as was apparent in the brief history of St Dymphna's. The unit at the Central Mental Hospital was administratively located within the forensic psychiatric system and offered a therapeutic programme, based on behaviourist 'token economy' principles, to small numbers of addicts transferred from Mountjoy Prison. The unit was staffed by male psychiatric nurses from St Brendan's Hospital, who had not been given any special training and who appear to have held extremely moralistic attitudes towards their charges. The inmates reciprocated by smuggling in large amounts of drugs through their weekend visitors and by generally challenging the legitimacy of the therapeutic system. The unit's medical director was quoted in 1975 as saying:

> We find that most of our patients, once they leave Dundrum, immediately take up their activities of abusing drugs again. In fact it seems to us that drug abusers in Dublin use all the treatment facilities more to avoid going to jail for their offences, or else to get lighter sentences in court, if they say they are undergoing treatment in Jervis Street, Usher's Island or Dundrum.[39]

The Usher's Island unit was opened in 1972 as an out-patient facility for young addicts. It was a well-staffed unit with a psychologist, a social worker and an occupational therapist as well as medical and nursing staff. As with the Dundrum unit, however, its staff appeared to become pessimistic quickly about its value and efficacy, and its psychologist was quoted in 1975 as saying that professional services, delivered in clinical surroundings, were less likely to be acceptable to young users than voluntary services staffed by young workers.[40]

By 1977, the year in which new comprehensive drugs legislation was enacted, both the Dundrum and Usher's Island services had been closed by the Eastern Health Board, leaving the Jervis Street service in a virtual monopoly situation. This failure of the Eastern Health Board to create and sustain a therapeutic response to illicit drug use and addiction within its psychiatric system was, of course, in marked contrast to the growing enthusiasm for alcoholism treatment which was evident, not just in the Dublin area but throughout the country, at this time. The reasons why there should be such a disparity between the development of alcoholism services and drug addiction services are worth exploring again before ending this section on treatment services. A study of the social and psychological characteristics of treated drug addicts in Dublin,[41] which was published in 1971, confirmed the accuracy of Fischer and Glanville's prediction that drug addicts would predominantly come from deprived urban areas, where drug use was part of a wider package of psycho-social problems, rather than being distributed randomly across socio-economic and geographic boundaries. As a patient group they appeared to have little to recommend them to the psychiatric services: they were truculent, unco-operative, and openly sceptical of the fundamental tenets of the psychiatric model of treatment; and, because of their poverty, they lacked the purchasing power to generate private treatment developments. No psychiatrist emerged to champion the cause of drug addicts and no national organisation comparable to INCA was formed to lend respectability to their cause. Perhaps the clearest and most explicit statement of disavowal on the part of the medical establishment was that contained in an editorial of the *Irish Medical Journal* in 1971, which said:

> The treatment of the established drug taker is extremely frustrating and therapeutically unrewarding. The task is usually given to our psychiatric colleagues. They can get patients successfully through the acute withdrawal phase which follows their admission to hospital and get them back to reasonable physical health. Subsequent management varies but psycho-therapy has not been demonstrably successful and psychiatrists are not willing to claim more than a very small percentage of cures ... One of the most heartening features of health care in Ireland over the last twenty years has been the great revival of voluntary effort in dealing with the handicapped members of society.[42]

The first, and for almost a decade the only, voluntary body concerned with the treatment of addicts in Dublin was Coolemine Therapeutic Community

which was set up in 1973.[43] The initiative for this development came from
Lord Paddy Rossmore, an Anglo-Irish peer who apparently had become
interested in drug problems as a result of seeing friends develop such
problems; financial support for the establishment of the Coolemine
residential facility came from the Eastern Health Board, from a range of
other statutory sources and from voluntary fund-raising. The concept of a
'therapeutic community' essentially consisted of utilising the entire social
milieu of residential facilities for the enhancement of the psychosocial
functioning of residents, rather than relying on the brief interventions of
psychiatrists or other professional therapists. The original therapeutic
community concept was the inspiration of a British psychiatrist, Maxwell
Jones, who experimented with this model of care for psychiatric patients,
starting in the late 1940s. The therapeutic community (commonly referred
to in drug treatment circles as the TC) model as applied to addiction
originated in the work of Charles Dederich, a recovering alcoholic who set
up a self-help foundation known as *Synanon* in 1958 at Santa Monica,
California.[44]

Unlike its British predecessor, the American TC for drug addicts was
based on a rigid hierarchical structure, with inmates moving up and down
the hierarchy as reward or punishment for their behaviour. The system as
a whole was based on the belief that addicts were immature, and the
treatment largely consisted of ritualised confrontation of this immaturity.
The Coolemine TC was introduced to Dublin through Phoenix House,
London, which was itself a creature of Phoenix House, New York.
Ideologically, the Coolemine programme was compatible with the general
rhetoric of drug treatment in Dublin during this period; it was assumed that
addicts had developed their drug habits because of individual personality
defects or deficits, and no causal significance was attributed to social
structural factors, such as unemployment, low income, poor housing or
communal demoralisation. The Coolemine programme consisted largely
of a self-help approach, and even its paid staff members tended to be
recovering addicts; this undoubtedly contributed to the credibility and
popularity of the service since – as in the case of Alcoholics Anonymous
– it was popularly believed that such personal experience of a drug
problem created a therapeutic advantage which professional training could
not match. For the first seven years of its existence, the Coolemine service
was very small, accommodating no more than nine clients in its residential
centre, and it was not until the major growth in prevalence of heroin use in
Dublin – from 1980 onwards – that it entered an expansionist phase.

In summary, it is clear that despite ministerial and other pronouncements
as to the value and desirability of providing treatment and rehabilitation
services for drug addicts, no service development comparable to that

which had occurred in the alcoholism field took place during this early period of Irish drug policy. In the Dublin area, which is where drug problems appeared to be most prevalent, the public psychiatric services displayed no interest in working with drug users and addicts, and instead one centralised service was developed at Jervis Street Hospital. The National Drug Advisory and Treatment Centre at Jervis Street received its funding directly from the Department of Health and, despite being based in Dublin and having a preponderance of Dublin patients, operated independently of the Eastern Health Board which was the statutory health authority for the Dublin area. Implicit in the overall pattern of treatment service development was the view that illicit drug users constituted a more deviant and behaviourally difficult client group than alcoholics; furthermore, it was assumed that the knowledge and skill base necessary for working therapeutically with these patients was highly specialised, so that it was pointless and possibly counterproductive to involve primary health care personnel in their treatment.

Misuse of Drugs Act, 1977

The Misuse of Drugs Bill, 1973 was published by the Minister for Health, Erskine Childers, in January 1973, only weeks before the Taoiseach, Jack Lynch, called a general election. Fianna Fáil, having been in government for the previous sixteen years, lost this election and was replaced by a coalition of Fine Gael and Labour. The change of government obviously complicated and delayed the debate on these legislative proposals, because it could not be presumed that the incoming Government would retain in its entirety the legislative proposals of its predecessor.

It was not until February 1975 that the new Minister for Health, Brendan Corish, took a somewhat amended version of the Misuse of Drugs Bill, 1973 into Dáil Éireann for its second reading. In his detailed introduction of the bill the Minister made what were coming to be customary remarks on the necessity to balance tough control systems with caring and humane treatment services:

> This is a complex bill which attempts to deal in a balanced way with a very complex problem. A tough approach on the question of criminality and unethical behaviour has been adopted, while at the same time I have attempted to meet the treatment and rehabilitation needs of drug abusers in a humane and enlightened manner.[45]

It would be untrue to say that in the ensuing debate nobody commented on the failure to develop treatment services; Charles Haughey, the Fianna Fáil spokesperson on health, wondered what progress was being made in setting up a residential detoxification unit at Jervis Street,[46] and Dr Hugh Byrne of Fine Gael expressed reservations about the Dundrum and Usher's Island facilities, besides commenting generally that 'people in the psychiatric services do not always percolate towards a fringe ailment like this'.[47] However, it would be equally untrue to say that the issue of treatment and rehabilitation became contentious or high-profile in this debate, or at any subsequent time during the passage of the bill through the Oireachtas.

The major Corish amendment to the earlier bill was contained in a new Section 28, which obliged the courts to defer sentencing of persons convicted under the main sections of the bill until medical and social reports were completed, and which also permitted the courts to commit such persons to a designated custodial treatment centre.

In general, however, the Misuse of Drugs Bill gave wide powers to the Garda Síochána to detain and search any person for whom there was 'reasonable cause' to suspect possession of the wide range of controlled drugs specified in the Schedule, and penalties for infringements of the bill – particularly for drug dealing – were tough. The second stage debate was lively and well-informed. Mr Haughey argued for the necessity to distinguish between 'hard' and 'soft' drugs, worried that increased police powers might erode civil liberties and wondered about the credibility of anti-drug legislation in a society which was so tolerant of alcohol and tobacco. Dr John O'Connell, a Labour TD at this time, also spoke at length; he disagreed with the presumption that cannabis was a dangerous drug which should be criminalised as it was in this bill, arguing that it was 'no more dangerous than a glass of beer'.[48] Significantly, most of the debate dwelt on the dangers which were assumed to be inherent in the drugs themselves and none of the speakers adverted to the causal link which might exist between socio-economic disadvantage and vulnerability to drug problems. There was, however, no evidence that the xenophobic view of Dr Hugh Byrne that all of Dublin's drug problems had their origins amongst foreign students at Trinity College Dublin was shared by other politicians.[49]

While the debate was lively, its tone was generally constructive and good-humoured, in sharp contrast with many parliamentary debates which are characterised by acrimony and political point-scoring. This is understandable because the topic was not one which readily lent itself to party political differences, and the bill being taken through the second stage by Mr Corish was essentially that which had been drafted by his Fianna Fáil predecessor. It was on this basis that the Minister for Health suggested that the third or committee stage of the Misuse of Drugs Bill, 1973 might be handled by a *real* committee, not by the whole Dáil acting in committee as was the norm at this time. Mr Corish had been at pains throughout to emphasise that he was open to all suggestions for improving the bill, and told the Dáil that he had 'asked Deputy Haughey if he would be agreeable to have it [the bill] sent to a special committee of the House where we could have a better discussion. There is no controversy about this Bill'.[50] Accordingly, a special committee consisting of fifteen Dáil deputies, and including three medical practitioners, was set up under the chairmanship of Barry Desmond of the Labour Party.

This committee met on fourteen occasions between October 1975 and June 1976 when it reported to Dáil Éireann on its proposals for amending the bill. The most significant change made by the committee was the abandonment of the Schedule system for categorising drugs, with cannabis being recognised uniquely as being less harmful by having lesser penalties attached for 'simple' possession. The debate at this committee in many ways reflected the earlier, second stage debate, with Dr Hugh Byrne protesting at what he saw as the folly of being soft on cannabis and Charles Haughey, in total disagreement, describing himself as 'reluctant to have any penalties for young people who fall into this particular social trap'.[51]

The report stage of the Misuse of Drugs Bill, 1973 did not take place until March 1977 and the bill then went to the Seanad in early May of that year, eventually becoming the Misuse of Drugs Act, 1977. The overall impression to be gained from reading the parliamentary debates on this piece of legislation is that the legislature was convinced that it had handled this subject in a reasonable and efficient manner. Ireland could now ratify the Single Convention on Narcotic Drugs 1961 and the Convention on Psychotropic Substances 1971, two United Nations conventions, and yet the legislature had avoided the worst excesses of societal over-reaction to this new and controversial social problem. The self-congratulatory tone of the legislature is succinctly captured in the words of Michael D. Higgins, then a Labour senator, who commented that:

> The point that has struck me most forcibly listening to this debate has been the difference between the debate in the Dáil and Seanad and the usual debate which takes place among the public on the subject of drugs and drug abuse. The public discussion is often insensitive and crude in a number of important ways.[52]

Conclusion

Whether or not such satisfaction with the state of Irish drug policy, and particularly with this legislation, was justified will become clearer over the next two chapters. Having achieved an early victory, in terms of securing the establishment of the Working Party on Drug Abuse, the informal networking activities of those closest to drug problems had to some extent been routinised through their incorporation into formal official structures, and it remained to be seen how effective this formal policy-making structure would prove to be. The Department of Health now played a lead role as co-ordinator of Irish drug policy and, as convenor and facilitator of the Inter-Departmental Committee on Drug Abuse (which included voluntary, statutory and professional interest groups), was expected to monitor the changing drug scene and plan for appropriate policy responses. An important, if somewhat unclear, role in the co-ordination of treatment services and the formulation of policy was also expected of the national Drug Advisory and Treatment Centre at Jervis Street Hospital, but the burden of direct service provision and the meagre resource allocation for this centre obviously raised questions as to the realism of these expectations.

By 1979, when the Misuse of Drugs Act, 1977 was brought into operation, there were already grounds for believing that the much vaunted balance between treatment and control was illusory; treatment services had not been developed and sustained within the Eastern Health Board service structures, and the liberal promise of Section 28 of the Misuse of Drugs Act, 1977 seemed doomed to failure because of the paucity of treatment and rehabilitation services. While it was asserted that drug issues represented the classic health promotional situation, where all sectors of government collaborated in a co-ordinated response, it also could be argued that the allocation of these issues to the Public Health Division of the Department of Health, rather than the Mental Health Division which ostensibly had responsibility for addiction treatment services, meant that even within the Department of Health there was no guarantee of balance or clear co-ordination on this subject.

Perhaps the most obvious and explicit policy complication which had arisen up to 1979 was that which concerned preventive drug education, yet it would have to be admitted that both the Working Party on Drug Abuse and the Committee on Drug Education handled the unexpected difficulties in this domain in a relatively sophisticated and efficient way. It was accepted that information-giving or admonitions not to use drugs – because drug use did not conform to our collective value systems – were unhelpful, and lifeskills approaches to health education were approved of as being most likely to succeed. However, the establishment of the Health Education Bureau as the agency to promote such lifeskills approaches meant that the Department of Health was no longer directly involved in this activity. There were valid reasons why the Department of Health, a policy-making body, should not become directly involved in the implementation of drug education programmes, but equally there were risks involved in assigning this task to a new and inexperienced agency should this policy become contentious.

Finally, no policy work was done on the possibility that the argument advanced by Fischer and Glanville (in their response to the draft education proposals of the Working Party on Drug Abuse) was correct, and that the major predictive factors in the Dublin drug scene would be socio-economic rather than individualistic. Irish drug policy, both in relation to drug education and treatment responses, remained resolutely individualistic, and the validity of this perspective was also to come under scrutiny in the period from 1980 onwards.

NOTES

1. H. Ghodse, 'International Policies on Addiction: Strategy developments and co-operation', *British Journal of Psychiatry,* 166 (1995), pp 14-18; K. Bruun, L. Pan and I. Rexed, *The Gentleman's Club: International Control of Drugs and Alcohol.* (University of Chicago Press, 1975); E. Nadelmann, 'Global Prohibition Regimes: the evolution of norms in international society', *International Organisation,* 144 (1990), pp 479-526.

2. J. Strang, 'The British System: past, present and future', *International Review of Psychiatry,* 1 (1989), pp 109-120; E. Schur, *Narcotic Addiction in Britain and America: the impact of public policy.* (London: Associated Book Publishers, 1966).
    The distinction between *maintenance* and *detoxification* should be clarified here. Detoxification refers to the process whereby an individual who is physiologically dependent on a drug is weaned off this drug under medical supervision, through the prescription of the drug or of a pharmacologically appropriate substitute. Maintenance, on the other hand, refers to the indefinite prescribing of an addictive drug where the prescriber is satisfied that the patient either cannot or will not remain drug free. The advantage claimed for maintenance is that the patient is treated with a clean and standardised pharmaceutical product and, secondly, that it offers an opportunity for a more socially stable and crime-free life.

3. *Report of the Working Party on Drugs Abuse.* (Dublin: Stationery Office, 1971), p.9.

4. *Report of the Commission of Inquiry on Mental Illness.* (Dublin: Stationery Office, 1966), p.84.

5. U. Macken, *Drug Abuse in Ireland.* (Cork: Mercier Press, 1975); S. Flynn and P.Yeates, *Smack: The Criminal Drugs Racket in Ireland.* (Dublin: Gill and Macmillan, 1985). Information on the early days of Irish drug policy presented here is based upon a number of informal discussions and one formal research interview with Denis Mullins, of the Garda Drug Squad. Noreen Kearney, a member of both the Working Party on Drug Abuse and the Committee on Drug Education, helped greatly by making available her papers from these committees and also by patiently answering innumerable questions and clarifying specific points.

6.   *Dáil Debates* (Vol. 243), Column 326.

7.   U. Macken, op.cit., p.84 (The quote is attributed simply to a 'lecturer in the College of Pharmacy in Dublin' but it is clear that this is Christy O'Connor).

8.   Interview with Joe O'Rourke, former Assistant Secretary at the Department of Health.

9.   *Report of the Working Party on Drug Abuse,* cit. sup., p.59.

10. Advisory Committee on Drug Dependence, *Cannabis.* (London: HMSO, 1968). The media and political response to this report is dealt with in J. Young, *The Drugtakers: the social meaning of drug use* (London: Paladin, 1971).

11. Personal communication from Dr Mullen.

12. *Report of the Working Party on Drug Abuse,* cit. sup., p.19.

13. Ibid, pp 14-15.

14. Ibid., p.52.

15. *Report of the Working Party on Drug Abuse,* cit. sup., p.59.

16. R. Wiener, *Drugs and Schoolchildren.* (London: Longman, 1970).

17. Letter from Professor E.F. O'Doherty to Tony O'Gorman (member of the Working Party on Drug Abuse), dated 5 June, 1970.

18. Letter from Rev. Patrick McDermott to Mary Whelan (member of the Working Party).

19. J. Naidoo, 'Limits to Individualism' in S. Rodmell and A. Watts (eds), *The Politics of Health Education: Raising the Issues.* (London: Routledge & Kegan Paul, 1986), p.17.

20. I. Fischer and B. Glanville, 'Education and Publicity on the Use and Abuse of Drugs' (Undated submission to the Working Party on Drug Abuse).

21. I. Fischer and B. Glanville, cit. sup., p.1.

22. Ibid., p.3.

23. Minutes of the 33rd Meeting of the Working Party on Drug Abuse held in the Conference Room (Department of Social Welfare) on Tuesday, 23 June, 1970.

24. *Report of the Working Party on Drug Abuse,* cit. sup., p.39.

25. *Report of the Committee on Drug Education.* (Dublin: Stationery Office, 1974), p.30.

26. Irish Council of Churches/Roman Catholic Joint Group on the Role of the Churches in Irish Society, *Report of the Working Group on the Abuse of Drugs* (1972), p.20.

27. S. Halleck, 'The great drug education hoax', *The Progressive,* 34 (1970), pp 1-7, cited in J. Swisher, 'Addiction Prevention – Future Directions', *Proceedings of Health Education Bureau Conference Education Against Addiction, 1979,* p.68.

28. *Report of the Committee on Drug Education ,* cit. sup., p.14.

29. Ibid., p.21.

30. The primary source for this account of the establishment of the Jervis St unit is: *Report on the Proposed Drug Addiction Clinic at Jervis Street Hospital,* an unpublished planning document drafted by Dr Joseph Woodcock, Honorary Secretary to the Jervis Street Hospital Medical Board; Dr John Ryan, Consultant Psychiatrist at Jervis Street; and Dr R.D. Stevenson, Consultant Psychiatrist, Dublin Health Authority. The account is also informed by many discussions of these events with Dr Stevenson.

31. *Report on the Proposed Drug Addiction Clinic Sited at Jervis Street Hospital,* cit. sup., p.2.
32. Ibid., p.5.
33. Ibid., p.3.
34. Ibid, p.4.
35. Ibid., p.5.
36. The proposal was to staff the Jervis Street Centre with one psychiatrist, two nurses and a social worker (*Report of the Proposed Drug Addiction Clinic Sited at Jervis Street Hospital,* cit. sup., 3).
37. *Report of the Working Party on Drug Abuse,* cit. sup., p. 41.
38. This account of the closure of St Dymphna's as a drug-treatment facility is based upon discussions with its clinical director, Dr Stevenson.
39. Cited in U. Macken, op. cit., p.100.
40. Ibid., p.103.
41. R. Stevenson and A. Carney, 'Social and Psychological Characteristics of Drug Addicts Interviewed in Dublin', *Irish Medical Journal,* 4 (1971), pp 372-375.
42. 'Care of the Drug Addict' (Editorial), *Journal of the Irish Medical Association,* 64 (1971), p.148.
43. Information on Coolemine and its origins is to be found in U. Macken, op. cit. and also in J. Comberton, *Drugs and Young People.* (Dublin: Ward River Press, 1982).
44. R. Janzen, *The Rise and Fall of Synanon: A California Utopia.* (Baltimore: Johns Hopkins University Press, 2001).
45. *Dáil Debates* (Vol. 278), Column 918.
46. Ibid., Column 933.
47. Ibid., Column 950-951.
48. Ibid., Column 967.
49. Ibid., Column 938.
50. *Dáil Debates* (Vol. 282), Column 375.
51. *Special Committee on the Misuse of Drugs Bill, 1973* (Minutes of Meeting of 10 December, 1975), p.50.
52. Seanad Debates (Vol. 86), Column 742.

6

Policy Responses to Dublin's Opiate Epidemic, 1980-1985

Introduction

The policy events described in Chapter Five appeared, on the face of it, to represent a solid list of achievements, marked by intersectoral co-operation and balance, and devoid of excessive moralism or hysteria. There was, however, to be a dramatic change in the drug scene in Dublin commencing in 1979/80, and this chapter will assess how the policies and structures set in place during the 1970s withstood the test imposed upon them by what came to be known as the 'opiate epidemic'.

A new style of drug use was first introduced to Dublin during the summer of 1970, consisting of the use of synthetic opiates – intended for oral consumption – which were ground down, mixed with a liquid and injected intravenously.[1] The drug most commonly used in this way was dipipanone (better known by its trade name *Diconal* or street name *dike*), a morphine alternative used conventionally for analgesic purposes. Apart from the risk of overdose associated with the use of this drug, there were the additional health risks associated with the introduction of contaminants into the bloodstream and with the sharing of unsterilised needles and syringes. While the practice of using this and other synthetic opiates in this way persisted, it did not apparently involve large numbers of drug users, nor did it lead to large-scale social and behavioural problems. A study of statistics referring to those charged with drug offences, contained in the Garda Commissioner's Annual Reports on Crime during the 1970s, does not suggest any real change in the pattern of illicit drug use, and it was ritually reported that 'cannabis continues to be the most widely used drug'.

However, a radical change occurred in the Dublin drug scene from 1979/80 onwards; this change involved the increased availability of heroin, which was now being 'pushed' for the first time on a commercial scale and was being used intravenously by increasing numbers of young people in some of the most disadvantaged inner-city and peripheral working-class neighbourhoods. In retrospect, it became apparent that the influx of relatively pure and cheap heroin into Ireland at this time was part of an international change in the pattern of drug trafficking, in which – for a variety of reasons – the 'Golden Triangle' area of South East Asia was replaced as the major exporter of natural opiates by the 'Golden Crescent' of Iran, Afghanistan and North-West Pakistan.

There are two major sources of official statistics which confirm this emergence of a heroin problem in Dublin, and the first of these, the Garda Commissioner's Crime Reports which have already been referred to, provides the data presented in Table 7.

Table 7: Heroin use as reflected by Garda crime statistics

Year	Total number of persons charged with drug offences	Number of persons charged with heroin offences	Quantities of heroin seized by with Gardaí (grammes)
1975	333	3	14 (+ 150 tablets) *
1976	289	–	1.6
1977	381	2	40 tablets *
1978	501	5	27.0
1979	594	5	5.0
1980	991	47	105.25
1981	1,256	177	170.134
1982	1,593	208	1,264.35
1983	1,822	449	1,279.04
1984	1,369	340	525.14
1985	1,270	359	1,220.0
1986	1,163	341	1,895.79
1987	1,196	256	51.56

* Information provided by Dr Desmond Corrigan of the School of Pharmacy, Trinity College Dublin, suggests that these heroin tablets contain 20 milligrammes of heroin. Thus 150 tablets would be the equivalent of 3 grammes of heroin, and 40 tablets the equivalent of 0.8 grammes of heroin. Although the Garda Crime Statistics do not make it clear, it is safe to assume that these quantities of heroin do *not* refer to pure heroin, but to the adulterated street drug which is of varying purity.

Source: Annual Reports on Crime by the Commissioner of the Garda Síochána to the Minister for Justice

Crime statistics must be interpreted with caution since they sometimes reflect changes in police activity or efficiency, rather than objective changes in criminal behaviour. The statistics referring to annual heroin seizures are a particularly good example of this need for cautious interpretation, since one or two big seizures will obviously have a major influence on the final annual statistic and yet may not be an accurate reflection of what is happening at street level. In 1986, for example, the total heroin seizure of 1,895.79 grammes was inflated by a single seizure of 1,311.60 grammes, involving an Italian national who was using Ireland as a transit point to her own country. Conversely, low heroin seizures by the police may sometimes conceal a flourishing street scene, albeit one which is fed by many couriers with small amounts of heroin rather than a few couriers with large consignments. Notwithstanding this *caveat,* it seems reasonable to infer from the data presented in Table 8 that there had been a major increase in the use of heroin and other drugs in the years following 1979. The Garda Drug Squad, which was still directed by Denis Mullins, fought its own battle for increased resources and in 1981 succeeded in having its numbers more than doubled. The health care response was somewhat slower to materialise although, as Table Six shows, the National Drug Advisory and Treatment Centre was treating significantly more drug users and particularly more heroin users.

Table 8: Numbers presenting for treatment at the National Drug Advisory and Treatment Centre, Jervis Street

Year	Total numbers of drug users	Numbers of heroin users (as % of all users)
1979	319	55 (17%)
1980	554	213 (38%)
1981	800	427 (53%)
1982	1,307	772 (59%)
1983	1,515	1,006 (66%)
1984	1,454	969 (67%)
1985	1,427	798 (56%)
1986	1,331	646 (48%)
1987	1,224	579 (47%)

Source: National Drug Advisory and Treatment Centre, Jervis Street

A number of local community groups also began to emerge in neighbourhoods where heroin use was perceived to be problematic; as part of their campaign for local prevention and treatment responses, these groups sometimes documented the scale of the heroin problem in their areas, and this community activism will be looked at later in the chapter. In general, the remainder of the chapter will assess the policy response to the so-called opiate epidemic from a health promotional perspective. It will ask whether the ongoing co-ordinated, intersectoral policy responses envisaged in Chapter Five proved to be a reality, and will also study the extent to which the health care authorities demonstrated a willingness and capacity to allow local communities to participate in defining the problem and in developing preventive and therapeutic initiatives.

Co-ordinating a national response

The first question that springs to mind in examining the policy response to the opiate epidemic is whether the Inter-Departmental Committee on Drug Abuse, which had been in existence since 1972, functioned effectively. The short answer to this question is that it did not, and that it failed to orchestrate a speedy response to the heroin problem; as will now be described in detail, there was no serious policy response to this changed situation until 1983.[2] Why this should have happened will also be explored. Because the Inter-Departmental Committee had no formal terms of reference, it was not obliged to meet on a regular basis to prepare reports for the Minister for Health, and it appears to have drifted into a pattern of sporadic meetings, with no coherent programme of work. When its abolition was mooted in 1983, it was suggested that it was this informal constitution and lack of specific terms of reference which had militated against the committee's effectiveness. However, as will be detailed below, some of its members have argued that the committee was never taken seriously by the Department of Health and was, in fact, thwarted by departmental officials.

By the time that heroin began to be readily available in 1979/80, Denis Mullins had been replaced on the Inter-Departmental Committee by a senior officer of the Garda Síochána who was only indirectly involved with drugs and who was unlikely to have had the same personal or professional commitment to this area of police work. However, three members of the committee (Martin Tansey of the Probation and Welfare Service; Joe Power of the Pharmaceutical Society; and Jim Comberton of the Coolemine Therapeutic Community) to whom this writer has spoken have insisted that the committee as a whole had fed detailed information on the changing drug scene and on the need for a vigorous policy response into the Department of Health. These informants were equally emphatic in their belief that the committee was never taken seriously by civil servants who tended to the view that reports of heroin problems were greatly exaggerated.

In any event, the Department of Health had still not publicly acknowledged by the end of 1981 that any change had occurred in the Dublin drug scene, nor had it attempted to introduce any new treatment or preventive measures. Media and political comment on the growth of a heroin scene had however begun to increase, and in November 1981 the Fianna Fáil spokesman on Justice, Gerry Collins, spoke at length on this topic in Dáil Eireann, concluding that 'Anybody who does not believe that the usage of heroin is growing has his head in the sand'.[3] Two weeks later it was reported in the *Irish Times* that the Pompidou Group of the Council of Europe had been told by Donal Creed, Minister of State at the Department of Health, and by Joe O'Rourke, Assistant Secretary at the Department of Health, that the heroin problem in Ireland had 'stabilised'.[4] In view of its previous failure to acknowledge that such a problem existed, this statement was greeted with anger and disbelief by community activists who were already involved in constructing 'bottom-up' responses to the heroin situation. Typical of these angry responses was a letter to the *Irish Times* from Barry Cullen, a community worker in the south inner-city, who argued that there were 'some communities in the Dublin area where even with the assistance of comprehensive treatment and rehabilitation resources, problems leading to and resulting from heroin dependency will now remain unsolved for decades'.[5]

In analysing the Department of Health's tardiness in reacting to this changed drug scene, it is again difficult to resist the conclusion that departmental officials at this time were poor 'networkers', who did not consult readily outside their own immediate circle or take seriously the views of those close to the drug scene, particularly when these views differed from some existing departmental view of their own. Ultimately the Inter-Departmental Committee appeared to become, in the words of Joe Power, just a 'talking shop' which met infrequently and had a mere token existence.

Barry Desmond, who was Minister for Health from November 1982 until January 1987, has argued retrospectively that departmental officials had no coherent view on this upsurge of heroin use, or on drug use generally, and that the Department of Health simply lacked the expertise and openness to analyse and respond to this new and complex medico-social problem. He also suggested that this administrative inertia was compounded by the political instability of this period, during which there were frequent changes of minister, thus strengthening the power of departmental officials.[6] The position of Minister for Health was subject to the following changes during these early years of the opiate epidemic:

• Charles Haughey was replaced by Michael Woods in December 1979.
• Michael Woods was replaced by Eileen Desmond in June 1981.
• Eileen Desmond was replaced by Michael Woods in March 1982.
• Michael Woods was replaced by Barry Desmond in November 1982.

It seems reasonable to conclude that a recognition of the need to develop some new policy initiative in response to heroin use was delayed by this inordinate turnover of Ministers for Health. It is also significant that this was a time of national economic difficulties, when increased health spending on drug prevention or rehabilitation would most likely be expected to come from the existing health budget rather than from additional funding; this economic reality must also have dampened the enthusiasm of Departmental officials for radical policy initiatives in this area.

The period from June 1981 to November 1982 was, as already stated, one of great political instability, involving three general elections. The short-lived Fianna Fáil Government of March to November 1982 was reliant on the electoral support of Tony Gregory, an independent TD from the north inner-city of Dublin, and amongst the various political favours and advantages which he sought for his constituency was a response to the heroin problem in this area. In general, local service providers and community activists from the north inner-city were highly incensed by the scepticism of Department of Health officials; the Department of Health was based in the Custom House at this time, so that civil servants were seen by residents of the north inner-city as ignoring a reality which was just outside their back door.

One important initiative taken by Michael Woods as Minister for Health was the commissioning of a prevalence study of drug use in the north inner-city. Although this study, which was started in September 1982 and finished in April 1983, could in many ways be seen as simply giving a scientific gloss to the statistics which local activists had already compiled, its findings and the publicity attaching to their presentation effectively led to drug issues being finally placed on the national policy agenda. The research was under the overall direction of Dr Geoffrey Dean, Director of the Medico-Social Research Board (MSRB); the senior researcher and author of the report was Dr John Bradshaw, and the field investigator was Fr Paul Lavelle who had served as Catholic Curate in the Seán MacDermott Street parish of the north inner-city.

The study, popularly referred to as the 'Bradshaw Report',[7] concluded that there was a ten per cent prevalence rate of heroin use in the 15-24 age group for the year prior to survey, while the rate was twelve per cent for the 15-19 age group and for girls in the 15-19 age group it was thirteen per cent. The study also showed that:

- eighty-four of the 88 heroin users (95 per cent) identified in the area were less than 24 years of age
- eighty-two (93 per cent) users said that they had been taking heroin at

least once a day, and 65 (74 per cent) said that intravenous use was
their preferred mode of use
- only four (4 per cent) identified users had any kind of educational
certificate, while 10 (11 per cent) were illiterate
- just four (4 per cent) of identified users were employed.

Understandably, these statistics were widely publicised by the media, as
was the report's conclusion that the Mountjoy A electoral area had a
prevalence of heroin use that was comparable with, and in some cases
worse than, some of the more notorious drug ghettoes in the United States.
The media did not, on the whole, pick up on the fact that the report had not
'demonised' heroin; that is, it had not portrayed heroin as being the sole or
primary corruptor of an otherwise functional social system. In fact,
Bradshaw discussed heroin use in this neighbourhood from a classic public
health perspective, seeing it not so much in terms of individual pathology,
but rather as being largely explicable in terms of adverse environmental
factors which struck him as self-evident. He expressed this conclusion in
stark terms:

> Finally, it is difficult not to think that these young people in North Central
> Dublin are the victims of society. They live in a dirty, squalid, architecturally
> dispiriting area; education seems to provide no mode of escape; unemployment
> is to be their almost inevitable lot; their parents are quite often separated or dead;
> abuse of alcohol is a common problem; crime the societal norm; imprisonment
> more likely than not; heroin taking is regarded as commonplace by quite young
> children; current treatment and rehabilitation facilities seem to hold little in the
> way of answers to their heroin abuse.[8]

The response of the Minister for Health, Barry Desmond, in the immediate
aftermath of the Bradshaw Report was to appoint a committee of six
Ministers of State under the chairmanship of Fergus O'Brien, Minister of
State at the Department of Health, to 'review and report on the question of
drug abuse, with particular reference to the Dublin inner-city area'.[9] This
committee, which was described as the *Special Governmental Task Force
on Drug Abuse,* had its first meeting on 28 April, 1983, and submitted a
report to Government during August of that year. The full report of this
Task Force was never published but many of its recommendations were
accepted by Cabinet and made public through a number of press releases
from the Department of Health on 20 September, 1983.

The decision to set up this committee of junior ministers, rather than a
more conventional expert committee, presumably reflected the
Government's sense of urgency as well perhaps as a fear that, in the
absence of direct political involvement, Department of Health officials

might continue to delay the formulation of new policy responses. In any event, the major recommendations of this Task Force which were publicly announced were the following:

- **Law enforcement:** The Misuse of Drugs Act, 1977 was to be amended to take account of the changed situation; there were also recommendations for improved policing and for streamlining judicial procedures in this area.
- **Treatment facilities:** It was recommended that the Jervis Street Centre be replaced by a purpose-built unit on the same site, and that in addition to having an in-patient detoxification unit at Beaumont Hospital (to replace the Jervis Street beds when Jervis Street Hospital closed, as it did in 1987), there should be a southside unit at St James's Hospital.
- **Education and research:** It was recommended that the MSRB should conduct further research into the prevalence of drug use and its social correlates, and that educational activities aimed at preventing drug use should be carried out both in high-risk areas and throughout society.
- **Community and youth development:** The Government recognised that drug abuse was both a 'youth problem' and one that was particularly common in deprived urban communities; it proposed, within existing budgets, to develop and co-ordinate a range of youth work and community development projects within the most vulnerable areas.

Collectively, these policy recommendations could be seen as incorporating all the main health promotion strategies, but it was the latter recommendation – on developments in community and youth work – which was potentially the most radical in its promise to recognise the causal importance of environmental factors. However, a careful reading of the full report of the Special Governmental Task Force on Drug Abuse *vis à vis* the various press releases on the unpublished report suggests considerable Governmental ambivalence on this topic, rather than an unequivocal abandonment of the traditional policy emphasis on individual pathology and individual vulnerability.

Section Four of the unpublished report contained a clear and explicit argument by its authors that the epidemic of drug abuse then being experienced in Dublin could be validly explained in terms of the poverty and powerlessness of the neighbourhoods concerned, rather than in terms of individual risk factors. The Task Force recommended that through the use of a number of indicators – prevalence of drug abuse, the crime rate, levels of educational attainment, the unemployment rate and the general state of social and recreational amenities – certain areas should be identified and designated as *Community Priority Areas* (CPAs). This designation would warrant the allocation of special, additional resources for job creation and training schemes, as well as the creation of new programmes designed to co-ordinate all existing statutory and voluntary social services in these areas. It was recommended specifically that each CPA should have within it a new body, to be called a 'Youth and Community Development Forum', which 'would draw up integrated plans for the provision and delivery of services and facilitate community responsibility for development'.[10]

The Task Force also recommended special funding for these CPAs: £500,000 to be allocated annually for all the CPAs, with a further £80,000 for the development of social and health education within the youth service sector, and a new 'Capital Grants Scheme for Community Facilities' which would have a budget of £500,000 for 1984.

These detailed recommendations for youth and community development as a means of drug abuse prevention never became known to the public because they were rejected at Cabinet and did not, therefore, feature in the press releases on the work of the Task Force issued on behalf of the Department of Health. No additional funding was provided and no new management structures were established to implement the summarised and by-now vague and aspirational recommendations on youth and community work contained in the press releases. It is difficult to know to what extent or how explicitly the Government considered this environmental or public health model of drug problems. The fact that youth and community issues were retained at all in the press releases suggests that this model was given some credence, but the traditional rhetoric of individualism was equally reflected in the Department of Health press releases. It was argued, for instance, that:

> The drug problem, which is mainly confined to the greater Dublin area, now affects young people particularly, without any reference to intellectual or educational attainment. No social class and no district in this area is exempt ... It cannot, however, be too strongly stressed that in this area, above all others, it is the individual decision which counts most.[11]

Barry Desmond has suggested that the decision to reject the Task Force's detailed recommendations on Community Priority Areas was based not so much on an ideological unwillingness to accept an environmental or public health model of drug problems, as on more mundane financial considerations and a belief that the Eastern Health Board and other relevant local authorities did not have the management capacity to create and sustain the inter-agency structures necessary to implement these recommendations.

Of the various recommendations made by the Special Governmental Task Force on Drug Abuse, it was those relating to law enforcement which were implemented most speedily and decisively, suggesting that supply reduction by vigorous enforcement of the criminal law continued to be the most uncomplicated and least uncomfortable policy response as far as the Government was concerned. Amended Misuse of Drugs legislation was introduced to the Oireachtas by Barry Desmond in early June 1984, and by August of that same year it had passed all stages, been signed by the President, and the commencement order for its implementation had been made. The major changes introduced by the Misuse of Drugs Act, 1984 may be summarised as follows:

- Penalties for drug offences were generally increased and the maximum sentence for drug trafficking was increased from fourteen years to life imprisonment.
- The mandatory requirement that judges should defer sentencing convicted drug offenders pending completion of medical and social reports (Section 28 of the Misuse of Drugs Act, 1977) was dropped.
- The definition of cannabis was altered to close off a legal loop-hole in the 1977 legislation.
- Drivers of motor vehicles and people in charge of boats or aircraft being searched for controlled drugs were compelled to remain with their vehicles for the duration of the search.
- It became an offence to publish, sell or distribute literature which advocated the use of controlled drugs.

If the parliamentary debate on the Misuse of Drugs Act, 1977 had been relatively liberal, perhaps reflecting the fact that Ireland had no serious drug problem at this time, the debate in 1984 was considerably less so. Politicians now seemed anxious to persuade the electorate that on the whole question of drug use and drug problems they were unequivocal and resolute, and despite the fact that it was the use of heroin which had necessitated this new legislation, a considerable part of the parliamentary debate was taken up with discussion of cannabis. Among the sources referred to by the Minister of State at the Department of Justice, Nuala Fennell, was a paper by Inspector John McGroarty of the Drug Squad entitled 'Cannabis: A Cultural Poison';[12] and in general the legislators concentrated on the evil which was deemed to be inherent in all illicit drugs, rather than on the socio-economic and other environmental factors which seemed to create vulnerability to serious drug problems among specific sub-groups of the population. Understandably perhaps, it appeared to be easier for the legislators to condemn the discrete evil of drugs, and the even more unspeakable evil of drug pushers, than to acknowledge the role played by unemployment, poverty and social deprivation generally in the creation of Dublin's opiate epidemic. While the language of Deputy Brendan McGahon was somewhat more extreme than that of most of his colleagues in the Oireachtas, his general views on this topic were not radically different from those of the majority of legislators. In the course of his contribution to the debate on the Misuse of Drugs Bill, 1984, Brendan McGahon said:

> Dependency on heroin is living death and the most extreme measures should be introduced to counteract it. Unfortunately, one of the drawbacks of a democracy is that it allows liberalism to flourish ... As far as drugs are concerned, liberals should not be allowed to be heard because surely nobody in his right senses can condone the taking of drugs, soft or hard. In other countries, drug pushers are dealt with summarily by being shot, and there is little or no drug pushing. I am not advocating that penalty here because it would not be accepted but, unfortunately, there will be commissions and inquiries and the problem will worsen and get out of control, as in the case of law and order.[13]

In Dáil Éireann an alternative perspective on heroin problems was articulated most clearly by Deputies Tony Gregory and Proinsias De Rossa, while in Seanad Éireann the policy thrust of the 1984 legislation was questioned most sharply and coherently by Senator Brendan Ryan. Among the issues which Brendan Ryan addressed was the alleged causal link between cannabis use and heroin use; his view on this was that, 'You have to do a little more than say because a person does two things, one follows from the other'.[14] He also quoted at length from a statement on the Misuse of Drugs Bill, 1984 which had been issued by the Irish Council for Civil Liberties (ICCL), which *inter alia* was critical of the proposals to make pre-sentencing medical and social reports discretionary. The ICCL had expressed concern that the new 'advocacy' offences, which prohibited publications which could be interpreted as promoting illegal drug use, might have the effect of stifling public debate on drug policy or might question the legality of any educational programme 'which admits as a matter of fact that pleasurable experiences can be obtained by the use of illegal substances'.[15] Finally, in his contribution to the debate on the Misuse of Drugs Bill, 1984, Brendan Ryan reiterated the views of Tony Gregory and Proinsias De Rossa concerning the causal link between heroin problems and social deprivation; as Brendan Ryan saw it, it would not be 'possible to deal with drug abuse on a universal scale or completely, if we leave areas of this city with dreadful housing, poor education and virtually no employment prospects'.[16]

In summarising this section, which has examined the way in which the

Government co-ordinated a national response to the upsurge of heroin use in Dublin from 1979/80 onwards, it must be concluded that the response was slow and, from a health promotional perspective, most unsatisfactory. The informal lobbying and networking activities which had been orchestrated by Denis Mullins in the late 1960s had been institutionalised by the establishment of the Inter-Departmental Co-ordinating Committee on Drug Abuse in 1972; much was expected of this latter committee but these expectations were largely disappointed. In its 1983 report, the Special Governmental Task Force on Drug Abuse accepted that the Inter-Departmental Committee had failed, and commented as follows:

> This Committee was established in 1972 so that those represented on it might exchange available information in relation to drug abuse which would enable deficiencies to be identified and effective action to be decided upon. However, it has been apparent for some time, particularly since the sudden dramatic rise in the incidence of heroin abuse in 1981, that the present Committee is not operating effectively. There are various reasons for this among which is the fact that the Committee was established on an informal basis without specific Terms of Reference. The members of the Committee are aware of these limitations and have been seeking additional powers for some time to enable them to exercise their functions effectively.[17]

This suggestion that the Committee's failure was attributable to its informal status and lack of specific terms of reference reflects a rather more disingenuous bureaucratic explanation than that which was advanced earlier in this section. Members of the Committee had suggested as an alternative explanation that the Department of Health had neither the will nor the capacity to co-ordinate policy development in relation to drug problems. The Inter-Departmental Committee, by virtue of its informal status, was almost totally dependent on the Department of Health and, it was argued, departmental officials took advantage of this situation to keep the Committee in an administrative limbo – much as they had done with the Working Group on the National Alcohol Policy, discussed in Chapter Four of this book. Looked at from a health promotional perspective, or particularly from an organisational networks framework, it seems as though the culture of the Department of Health encouraged its officials to look inwards and to treat with scepticism any externally-generated information, ideas or policy recommendations which did not coincide with their own conventional wisdom on drug problems. Members of the Committee who tried to persuade the Department of Health that a major change had occurred in the Dublin drug scene, reported that this message was treated with polite disbelief: the Department was unconvinced that any serious change had occurred and appeared to believe that its main duty was to prevent any policy over-reaction in this area. The recommendation of the Special Governmental Task Force on Drug Abuse on this matter was that a new National Co-ordinating Committee on Drug Abuse, with specific terms of reference, should be established to replace the Inter-Departmental Committee which had been in existence since 1972. The new committee did not come into being until 1985 but by tracking its progress (this will be done in Chapter Seven) thereafter it should be possible to throw further light on these alternative explanations as to why the co-ordinating structure – of which there were such high hopes – failed to live up to expectations.

Prevention and treatment – collaboration between local communities and statutory services

The events and issues to be discussed here are, potentially at least, the very stuff of health promotion. A serious heroin problem had emerged in Dublin, and there was evidence that it was not distributed randomly but that it was linked to socio-economic deprivation and was confined to identifiable communities. An important question which this posed for health authorities was whether they would acknowledge the importance of these environmental factors and work collaboratively with the communities most affected, or whether they would continue with a more traditional biomedical approach to heroin use and heroin addiction. Such a biomedical approach would involve the provision of treatment and rehabilitation by professional health-care workers, based on an individualistic model, and probably delivered from central rather than local services and facilities. A health promotional or public health response, on the other hand, would consist of close collaboration between health authorities and affected communities, based on an acceptance of the causal importance of environmental factors, and involving members of the community and primary care personnel in the delivery of locally-based services. Referring back to the Ottawa Charter which has identified five main tasks considered essential to the realisation of health promotion, the following three tasks are particularly relevant to the analysis of health service responses to the opiate epidemic:

• **Creating supportive environments** – this would involve the health authorities in recognising that both the physical and social environments of some Dublin neighbourhoods were generally inimical to good health and were specifically contributing to a high incidence and prevalence of heroin problems

- **Strengthening community action** – this would involve the health authorities in the creation of participative structures and processes whereby local residents might actively collaborate in defining the problems of their communities and putting together both preventative and therapeutic responses to these problems
- **Reorienting health services** – this is little more than a summarised statement of the necessity for health authorities and professionals to move from their previous preoccupation with curative matters to a holistic approach which would recognise the importance of environmental factors, accept the validity of lay knowledge and lay participation in health-care matters, and also acknowledge the valuable role of primary care health care workers.

It will be recalled from Chapter Five that during the period from the mid-1960s to the late-1970s the Dublin Health Authority and its successor the Eastern Health Board had not developed any real treatment system for those using or dependent upon illicit drugs. No independent lobby group had emerged to argue the case for such treatment systems and, unlike the situation pertaining to alcohol problems, there appeared to be no enthusiasm on the part of psychiatrists to become involved with the treatment and rehabilitation of illicit drug users. Furthermore, the creation of the National Drug Advisory and Treatment Centre at Jervis Street Hospital as a 'stand-alone' facility had made it unclear whether there was any necessity for the Eastern Health Board to develop its own services for drug users.

In 1979, however, the Eastern Health Board made an internal management decision which, on the face of it, had interesting and important implications for its future management of illicit drug problems. This was the decision to transfer responsibility for drug problems from the Board's Special Hospital (Mental Health) to its Community Care Programme. This transfer of responsibility could be interpreted as signalling a new policy orientation, acknowledging the reluctance of the psychiatric services to become involved with drug users and the perceived desirability of developing localised prevention and treatment initiatives. McKinsey, the management consultants who had designed the management structures of the health boards following the Health Act, 1970, had argued that the Community Care Programme could be expected to deliver services which were 'community based, where local knowledge and insight is of great assistance to their efficient administration and where constant communication and contact with the local population is essential'.[18] If the transfer of drug problems into the administrative sphere of Community Care resulted in the application of this philosophy to drug problems, then it could certainly be said that health promotion was being taken seriously in this field.

The truth of the matter, however, was that the motivation underlying this change was more mundane and, from a policy perspective, more disappointing than this. What happened, quite simply, was that a Senior Administrative Officer in the Board's Special Hospital Programme transferred as a personal career move to Community Care and it was decided that 'she should take drugs with her'.[19] At the time of her transfer, it became apparent to senior management in the Eastern Health Board that this officer was – by virtue of almost ten years experience of dealing with drug issues – the only senior administrator in the organisation who could be regarded as having any expertise in this field. The Board could have decided to take this opportunity to insist that the psychiatric services take a more active and responsible role in relation to illicit drugs or alternatively, it could have reviewed the whole topic from a Community Care perspective and set up formal management or policy-making structures to incorporate drug services into Community Care. It did neither in fact, but rather than seeing this as something that demanded reflection and careful policy formulation, opted to regard the management of drug problems as a discrete and uncomplicated administrative matter best left with the individual officer who had previously handled it.

Even nine years after this event, when this writer discussed the transfer of drugs to Community Care with Michael Walsh, then Programme Manager for the Special Hospital Programme, Mr Walsh did not see this event as unusual or questionable.[20] Áine Flanagan, the administrator in question, was reluctant to speak at length on this subject, other than to reject the suggestion that the Board's transfer of drug issues to Community Care reflected any policy view on this matter; it was, she suggested, another example of what she termed Health Board 'ad hoccery'.[21]

The significance of all this is that, just as Dublin was about to experience a dramatic increase in opiate use, the Eastern Health Board had neither a formal management structure to deal with this problem nor any coherent view as to what its role should be in relation to this problem. It displayed no self-critical or reflective capacity in this regard, seeing the drugs issue as one which could largely be left to the discretion of a single administrator rather than one which called for on-going policy formulation. This placed Áine Flanagan in an invidious position; she was, it would generally be agreed, an intelligent, formidable and hard-working administrator but, lacking either specific professional training or a clear policy line to guide her in the complex arena of Dublin's heroin problem, she was largely reliant on her own instincts as to how best to respond. These instincts, it should be remembered, had been developed and honed in a traditional clinical model of service provision, where the 'authorities' set up systems for healthcare professionals to treat a relatively passive laity, rather than in any form of participative community work.

Before looking in some detail at a number of case-studies of community responses to the heroin problem, reference will first be made to the *Task Force on Drug Abuse* which was set up in the late summer of 1982 within the Eastern Health Board, and which represented the Board's only formal attempt at policy making on this topic during this period. This Task Force was set up by the Chief Executive Officer of the Eastern Health Board with the following terms of reference:

> To examine and quantify the extent of drug abuse in the Eastern Health Board area, to recommend appropriate action in the prevention and treatment area to deal with the problem and to co-ordinate such activity within the Eastern Health Board area.[22]

The Task Force was chaired by the Director of the Eastern Health Board's Forensic Psychiatric Service, Dr Liam Daly, and in addition to other representation from the Board, its members included personnel from Jervis Street, the Departments of Health, Education and Justice, the Health Education Bureau, Coolemine Therapeutic Community and the Garda Drug Squad (which was still represented by Denis Mullins).

In view of the reluctance of Eastern Health Board psychiatrists to become involved with drug users, the decision of the EHB's Chief Executive Officer to appoint a psychiatrist as chairman of this Task Force may be seen as indicative of the vague and confused approach which its management generally had towards drug issues, and it appears that much of the responsibility for managing the Task Force and producing a report fell upon Áine Flanagan. Ms Flanagan herself described the workings of the Task Force as 'half-hearted', and suggested that in the circumstances she felt obliged to take a leadership role. Her behaviour in doing so left her open to criticism from others, such as Jim Comberton of Coolemine Therapeutic Community, who felt that his viewpoint was not taken into consideration during this process.[23] A similar criticism was made by Paul Harrison, an Eastern Health Board social worker, who also thought that this Task Force was a missed policy opportunity on the part of his employing organisation.[24]

The report of the Task Force offered little by way of comfort for those who might have hoped for evidence of a clear strategy on drugs on the part of the Eastern Health Board. It was a poorly written and confused document, consisting of just five pages of discussion and recommendation, followed by 50 pages of appendices. The recommendations are not spelt out clearly, do not flow logically from the preceding text and do not focus on activities which were specifically within the remit of the Eastern Health Board. The report is best regarded as a non-event, and from a policy analysis perspective it is perhaps more illuminating to point out what it did *not* do. It did not:

- focus upon the almost total abdication by the public mental health services in Dublin of all responsibility for drug problems
- attempt to clarify the working relationships, or division of labour, between the National Drug Advisory and Treatment Centre (Jervis Street) and the Eastern Health Board
- clearly identify heroin as the drug which was causing the most social and behavioural disruption in Dublin at this time
- acknowledge the localised nature of heroin problems in specific neighbourhoods, or attempt to produce policy guidelines for collaborative work with the residents and primary care personnel of these areas.

It was pointed out in Chapter Five that the establishment of the National Drug Advisory and Treatment Centre at Jervis Street Hospital had been modelled on the British policy decision to locate drug treatment services in centralised facilities, which were colloquially referred to as 'the clinics', run by specialist staff. The wisdom and practicality of this policy came under scrutiny in the early 1980s when Britain, like Ireland, experienced a dramatic increase in opiate use. In December 1982, the Advisory Council on the Misuse of Drugs, Britain's statutory drugs advisory body, published its *Treatment and Rehabilitation* report which argued that it was no longer practicable to expect all problem drug takers to be treated by specialist staff in centralised clinics; instead, it recommended that local drug services should be established which would largely be reliant on the contribution of generic primary health and social service personnel.[25] It would be unfair to suggest that the Eastern Health Board's Task Force should have considered this influential British report, because *Treatment and Rehabilitation* was published just as the Task Force was completing its own report. It would not be unfair, however, to say that the issues involved – the relative merits of centralised and local services – were reasonably obvious, and that its failure to address them confirms the Task Force's lack of analytic capacity.

While it is difficult to draw definite conclusions from the brief and meandering text of the Task Force report, what appears to come across is that its authors were unconvinced about the gravity of this upsurge in heroin use. Specifically, it appears that the Task Force was insensitive to the needs of those neighbourhoods where heroin use was creating new and seriously disruptive social problems, directly involving very young drug users and indirectly involving entire communities. It was argued that 'The problem, in terms of damage to the region's health, from the "Abuse of Drugs" is still relatively small, particularly when it is compared with the wider effects of cigarette smoking and alcoholism'.[26] This point is valid only in terms of crude, total population indicators, but, as the Bradshaw Report was confirming at this time, more specific indicators based on the study of cohorts of young people in inner-city neighbourhoods showed a very different picture for those who lived in these neighbourhoods.

Health Board / Community collaboration: three case-studies

The material considered in this section refers to three working-class areas of Dublin which were particularly affected by the opiate epidemic: the areas in question are St Teresa's Gardens in the south inner-city, the Seán MacDermott Street area of the north inner-city and Ballymun, a peripheral high-rise development to the north of the city which had been built in the 1960s. It will be shown that what happened in each of these areas by way of response to heroin problems can be seen as approximating to the *organisational networks* style of policy making discussed in Chapter One. In other words, this response to heroin problems was neither of the *rational-comprehensive* type, involving the State in a top-down and co-ordinated plan, nor of the *partisan mutual adjustment* type, consisting of an incremental process of bargaining and compromise between all the interest groups involved; instead, the response to heroin problems in these three communities evolved from the on-going relationships between local representatives of various human service organisations and indigenous community leaders.

   In view of the controversy and the allegations of violence, vigilantism and political subversion which were to be made against some of the later anti-drugs groups, it is important to emphasise how 'respectable' and mainstream these original community networks were.[27] In the Ballymun area, for example, a local resident, Queenie Barnes, became concerned in late 1980 at the prevalence of heroin use and, following the deaths of three young people from drug-related causes, she approached Ineke Durville, an Eastern Health Board Community Care social worker for the area. The groundwork for the establishment of the Youth Action Project was carried out in early 1981 by these two people and by Frank Deasy, a social work student from Trinity College Dublin on placement with Ineke Durville. In the Seán MacDermott Street area, similarly, the initiative for developing specific anti-drug measures in the area came in 1981 from an informal social service group, the 'V & S', so-called because it was made up of both voluntary and statutory social service personnel. This group involved, amongst others, Paul Harrison, a Community Care social worker with the Eastern Health Board, and Fr Paul Lavelle, the local Catholic Curate. In St Teresa's Gardens the anti-drugs initiative stemmed largely from the Eastern Health Board's community care social work post which had been in existence since 1972 and which – through a succession of holders of this post – had created a good working relationship with a local residents' group, the St Teresa's Gardens Development Committee. As early as 1980, this group was convinced of the necessity to provide a local response to the growing use of heroin, and in 1981 a specific community group called the Youth Development Project (YDP) was established to combat the heroin problem. At the end of 1981 the committee of the YDP consisted of the following:

> Dr Fergus O'Kelly, General Medical Practitioner
> Fr Seán McArdle, Catholic Curate
> Patricia Smith, Probation and Welfare Officer
> Matt Bowden, Secretary of the St Teresa's Gardens Development Committee
> Michael King, Principal of Liberties Vocational School
> Barry Cullen, Social Worker, Eastern Health Board
> Paul Humphrey, Chairperson of the St Teresa's Gardens Development Committee
> Ray Kavanagh, Assistant Section Officer, Community Care Programme, Eastern Health Board
> Sam Anglin, Coolemine Therapeutic Community

It is clear that this committee was almost entirely made up of conventional caring service personnel rather than of political subversives eager to exploit the emerging heroin crisis in St Teresa's Gardens; indeed if any criticism were to be made of its make-up, it would probably be that local residents were under-represented on it.

Having established who was involved in these local networks, it is equally important to clarify what their views were and what vision they had for the eradication of heroin problems from their areas. While there may have been subtle differences between the three groups being considered here, by and large they developed a common vision which may be described as health promotional in its essence. In summary, these local networks may be seen as making three points:

- that there was a big increase in heroin use amongst the young people in these areas and that this new form of drug use was leading to unprecedented health and social problems
- that this prevalence of heroin use was causally linked to the poverty and the communal demoralisation which characterised these areas

• that treatment and preventive measures could not be delivered in a traditional biomedical way, with an emphasis on expert therapists treating pathological individuals, but that a social and participative model must be established at local community level.

This vision was expressed with varying degrees of clarity and conviction to the Eastern Health Board, the Department of Health and Dublin Corporation. Some of the analysis was extremely detailed and explicit, as, for example, in the submission of Barry Cullen to the Lord Mayor of Dublin in October 1981; it had been proposed to establish a working party on drug use within Dublin Corporation and, with the agreement of his Director of Community Care, Barry Cullen submitted a document to the Lord Mayor, setting out the agenda and philosophy of the group then working in St Teresa's Gardens. Having made the point that it was heroin use which had caused this group to come into existence, Barry Cullen went on:

> People from all backgrounds, experiences and situations will come in contact with drugs; some will use and become addicted to them. This is a human reality. However, and this point is fundamental to understanding Dublin's drug problem, the widescale use of hard drugs can only be a major problem for a particular community, it can only be endemic to that community, when the social, economic and environmental conditions allow it ... When social and economic planners deny urban communities a role in planning their own development, they are predisposing such vulnerable communities to a hard drug problem.[28]

This perspective on drug problems is, of course, similar to that enunciated by Fischer and Glanville in their submission to the Working Party on Drug Abuse (discussed in Chapter Five) but its implications for prevention and treatment were profoundly at odds with the biomedical perspective that had implicitly underpinned all drug treatment and rehabilitation in Dublin up to this point. At its most radical, this bottom-up model of drug problems called for major restructuring of local governmental systems in the areas in question, with local residents being afforded a much greater opportunity to participate in housing policy and in other social and environmental services, as well as in training and job creation schemes. At a less radical level, this new vision of drug problems insisted that it was no longer acceptable that treatment service provision should be located in centralised facilities – at a geographic remove from the communities most afflicted – dominated by healthcare professionals. Two years after its foundation, the Ballymun Youth Action Project summarised its philosophy in the following way:

> In this approach, we see the primary problem facing the individual abuser and
> his/her family as one of addiction and seek to develop community based
> supports. In terms of the wider community we seek to develop the awareness,
> skills and resources necessary to cope with and prevent the escalation of drug
> abuse as a community problem.[29]

In terms of practical politics, the main demand being made of the Eastern
Health Board, therefore, was for the establishment of community-based
counselling and rehabilitation facilities and youth work services, in which
local residents and locally-based professionals could work collaboratively
with the Health Board. The fundamental difficulty which the Health Board
had with this demand was that, as discussed in relation to its Task Force on
Drug Abuse, it did not appear to be fully convinced that a serious drug
problem existed and therefore did not accept the necessity for reviewing or
changing existing service provision. The first task of the local drugs
groups was, therefore, to persuade the Eastern Health Board that a heroin
problem actually existed, and this will now be looked at in some detail.

The frustration and anger of local community activists at official
scepticism, was graphically illustrated in a paper written by Willie Martin,
a voluntary community worker in St Teresa's Gardens during this period.
He wrote:

> By that summer of 1983, the use of heroin had reached epidemic proportions in
> the city of Dublin. St Teresa's Gardens was one of the worst affected areas. It was
> estimated that over 200 junkies a week were getting their supply of heroin in St
> Teresa's Gardens. The flats were in a constant upheaval of vomit, urine, blood and
> overdoses. Many of the junkies were so badly in need of a vein to fix into that they
> pulled down their pants and searched their lower parts, not giving a damn about
> the children who would be passing up and down the stairs ... For years we had
> been struggling to alleviate the problem but with little success. It was not our fault.
> We had approached all the right people – Ministers for Health, TDs, Corporation
> officials and the police. Nobody took us seriously. They implied that if there was
> a drug problem wouldn't they be the first to know about it.[30]

In St Teresa's Gardens and in Seán MacDermott Street the local anti-drugs
groups had engaged in what may be described as 'popular epidemiology'
in an attempt to persuade the Department of Health and the Eastern Health
Board that their communities were experiencing a new and unprecedented
wave of heroin use. Popular epidemiology is an American concept which
refers to the way in which ordinary citizens and primary care personnel –
as opposed to specialist healthcare professionals – gather data and present
the authorities with their findings in support of their convictions that their
communities are experiencing environmental health problems.[31] The
'experts', in this case the Department of Health, the Eastern Health Board

and the National Drug Advisory and Treatment Centre at Jervis Street, had not accepted that heroin use had increased as radically or as destructively as the local groups perceived it to have, so the local groups set about researching and documenting their case as systematically as they could.

The first research of this kind, which consisted of a pooling of information gathered by local residents and locally-based professionals, was carried out in October 1981 by the St Teresa's Gardens group and later submitted to the Eastern Health Board. Its main findings were that:

- of 350 families in the target area, 40 had at least one member who was a heroin user
- 57 heroin users were identified in this community, 39 of whom were over the age of 18, and 18 of whom were in the 12-18 age group
- the number of children deemed to be 'at risk' by virtue of residence with a heroin user was 35
- the youngest heroin user identified by the researchers was 12 years old and it was estimated that he had been using heroin for two years at the time of the survey.

The Seán MacDermott group used a similar methodology during 1982 to calculate the prevalence of heroin use in its own area, and when some of its members met the Minister for Health in May 1982 they reported that in their area there were 50-60 heroin users between 12 and 18 years of age. It is at this point that the political issues surrounding this form of popular epidemiology become obviously pointed. It appears that both EHB and Department of Health officials remained unconvinced about the validity of these prevalence figures and of the necessity for taking decisive action in relation to heroin; in this circumstance, the Minister (Dr Michael Woods) decided that the health care system would only respond when there was 'scientific' evidence to this effect, and he accordingly commissioned prevalence studies from the Medico-Social Research Board. This led to the completion and publication of the Bradshaw Report, referred to earlier in this chapter. The Seán MacDermott group co-operated fully with the Medico-Social Research Board, and the main investigator in their area was, as previously mentioned, the local curate Fr Paul Lavelle. The YDP Committee of St Teresa's Gardens met Dr Bradshaw but refused to co-operate with the research which he and Dr Geoffrey Dean of the Medico-Social Research Board proposed to carry out in their area. Cullen, in discussing the YDP's motives for not co-operating with Bradshaw, has said:

> The committee discussed this matter and having considered what were now obvious political dimensions to Bradshaw's second phase study, and for other

reasons – particularly their concern that a comprehensive survey would raise local expectations that an official response was imminent – refused to participate any further in the study. Furthermore, members of the committee expressed strong views that the information collected to date, and submitted already to the health board was sufficient to warrant a substantial official response and that little was to be gained, at this stage, by participating in further research.[32]

The publication of the Bradshaw Report received considerable publicity, with which some residents of the north-inner city were unhappy, claiming that it merely gave the area an even worse name than it already had.[33] While it may have led directly to the setting up of the Special Governmental Task Force and indirectly to the enactment of the Misuse of Drugs Act, 1984, the Bradshaw Report did not lead to clearer or more harmonious relationships between the Eastern Health Board and the local groups which were concerned with heroin problems in these areas.

At their meeting with the Minister for Health in May 1982 the Seán MacDermott group had presented the Minister with detailed plans for a local service. It was reported to the Eastern Health Board that 'The delegation said they already have a site – the Youth and Community Centre – which could be used as a walk-in treatment centre for young addicts. They need professional staff. They also want to be involved themselves in the centre to encourage young people to come in.'[34] Following this meeting the Minister approved a grant of £20,000 towards the cost of setting up this local centre, and in August 1982 Paul Harrison, an Eastern Health Board Community Care social worker, was appointed as Project Leader to the centre. However, the working relationship between the local group and the Eastern Health Board quickly became strained and acrimonious. The perception of the local group was that the Eastern Health Board did not want to develop any drug project in which it had to share power with local residents and locally-based professionals, but that it was only comfortable with a conventional treatment model – namely one which was run by professionals and managed by the Health Board. After five months in his post as Project Leader, convinced that his own employing organisation (the Eastern Health Board) would commit itself neither philosophically nor financially to the proposed new service, Paul Harrison resigned from his post and went back to Community Care social work. A treatment centre for young drug users was in fact established in the north inner-city during 1983, but it was directed by a social worker who had previously worked in the National Drug Advisory and Treatment Centre, Jervis Street and it developed as a professionally-run, centralised service with minimal local connections.

A very similar set of events took place in St Teresa's Gardens where the local YDP had developed detailed and elaborate proposals for a locally-based treatment centre for young drug users. The Eastern Health Board initially agreed to collaborate with the YDP in the establishment of this centre but, as in the case of the Seán MacDermott project, this agreement was followed by increasingly bitter exchanges between the two parties. The first Project Leader appointed to the St Teresa's Gardens venture, Helen Walker, also resigned after a short period in office, mirroring the motivation and actions of Paul Harrison in the north inner-city. She was replaced by Barry Cullen, another Health Board social worker, but, after what resembled a war of attrition, it became clear that the Eastern Health Board would not participate in the proposed new centre and the plan came to nothing.

In Ballymun, the YAP had evolved slowly and had not produced detailed proposals for a new treatment centre or made serious financial demands on the Health Board. In 1983 it employed Mary Ellen McCann, an experienced addiction counsellor, to work for it on a half-time basis; she was the organisation's first paid worker, and it was not until late 1984 that a grant from the Youth Affairs Section of the Department of Labour allowed it to advertise for its first full-time post. Within days of this post being advertised, however, the YAP discovered that the Eastern Health Board had appointed an addiction counsellor to work in Ballymun; this appointment caused great annoyance to YAP which believed that it should have been consulted, or at least informed, about this development. The ensuing row, in early 1985, received newspaper coverage which publicly and explicitly highlighted the disagreements between the Health Board and local groups as to what constituted 'community care' for young drug users. In the course of a long letter to the *Irish Times,* members of YAP said:

> The [Eastern Health] Board's statement that they are interested in working together would be more credible if this had been a joint decision. Far from helping our project to develop, this leaves us with a new set of circumstances to deal with – what are the Health Board plans for the area? Are local people to be totally excluded from those plans? *How* are we supposed to work together? ... It would seem there are perceptions of what constitutes resources being 'community-based'. Those caught in the middle of those differences are those most in need of help – addicts and their families.[35]
> (Italics as in original)

A fuller account of this debacle is contained in *Ten Years On,*[36] the history of the YAP which was written when the project was ten years old, but the YAP perception of these events essentially corresponds to that of the St Teresa's Gardens and Seán MacDermott Street groups: the Health Board was seen as being unwilling or unable to share power with local groups in creating a response to drug problems.

The World Health Organisation, as described in Chapter One, had published its *Strategy for Health for All by the Year 2000* in 1978 and had continued to develop these health promotional ideas thereafter. A 1985 WHO publication which sought to define specific targets for its *Health for All* programme argued that:

> It is a basic tenet of the health for all philosophy that people must be given the knowledge and influence to ensure that health developments in communities are made not only for but also with and by the people.[37]

The anti-drug activities described in this section could be seen as exemplary of health promotion at community level, yet the Eastern Health Board consistently appeared to resent and thwart these developments. In seeking to understand this, there are a number of plausible explanatory factors which suggest themselves. The first such explanation, which has already been touched upon, concerns the lack of policy discussion of any issues at both Department of Health and Health Board levels. No real debate had taken place at a high policy level in relation to illicit drugs, and the only ideas which guided Irish policy in this area were the minimalist and rather superficial ideas contained in the *Report of the Working Party on Drug Abuse* (1971). Had this committee given credence to the Fischer and Glanville submission on the importance of socio-economic factors in the causation of drug problems, this might have facilitated the Eastern Health Board in linking abstract ideas about health promotion and community care to the concrete bottom-up initiatives in working-class communities described here.

In the absence of formal debate on drug issues at central government level or the creation of dedicated management structures at EHB level, a great deal of discretion lay with Áine Flanagan who, as the senior administrator dealing with drug issues within the EHB, carried almost total responsibility for the Board's response to the opiate epidemic. It has already been acknowledged that Ms Flanagan was in an unusual and invidious position, and it is important in discussing these events that she should not be personally criticised in any way, but rather seen as representing the administrative system of the time to which she belonged. Furthermore, as will become clear later in this section and in Chapter Seven, there are problems and disadvantages attaching to community participation in drug treatment services which may be seen as justifying EHB scepticism in this matter. It is relatively easy to understand Áine Flanagan's motives and intentions in this matter, however, since she was always quite forthright in explaining and defending Health Board activities.[38]

Stated simply, Áine Flanagan had major reservations about the concept of community work or community development in the sense that this implied a participative element to health and social service provision as reflected, for example, in the WHO statement quoted above. Instead, her vision consisted of a traditional approach to service delivery, in which the planning and administration of services were carried out by health authorities (such as the Health Board) with the services then being delivered by professionals; the role of service consumers in this traditional view was, of course, a relatively passive one, with little or no credence being given to the idea that lay people had any wisdom to contribute to service planning or delivery. Ms Flanagan was critical of Health Board employees who became integrated into local networks, and took the view that loyalty to the Health Board should take precedence over other loyalties which might arise locally. Insofar as she understood the WHO concept of community empowerment she disapproved of it, believing that treatment services could be delivered more effectively by professionals and that service provision could be damaged by community involvement. Implicitly her view of power was of the zero-sum type: the more power a local community group acquired, the less power was left for the Health Board.

The administrative culture of the Eastern Health Board's Community Care Programme at this time appeared to be one which did not, in the main, value formal planning or analysis.[39] Officers of the Board appeared to see their own viewpoint as reflecting their hard-won experience and administrative commonsense, and such beliefs tended not to be recorded in written form but to be retained and passed on anecdotally as part of an oral tradition. No mechanisms existed whereby the policy statements and plans of community groups could be considered as part of a formal planning process within the Health Board, and officers did not appear to appreciate how difficult it was for outside bodies to understand the Health Board's position in the absence of clearly written policy statements.

From 1983 onwards, the Eastern Health Board built up a network of community-based addiction counsellors who were expected to undertake therapeutic work with addicts and their families. This addiction counselling was organised along conventional therapeutic lines – it was almost entirely individualistic in orientation and took little or no account of the wider socio-economic environment – and the intention was that it would be supervised from Jervis Street.

Throughout this period, the National Drug Advisory and Treatment Centre at Jervis Street continued to have a monopoly in terms of the medical assessment, detoxification and rehabilitation of drug users. Media and public opinion of Jervis Street throughout the period of the opiate epidemic appears to have been uniformly positive, with much sympathy being expressed for the poor facilities and general lack of resources which were the lot of the centre's staff. In 1983, Peter Murtagh of the *Irish Times* described the Jervis Street premises as an 'undercapitalised slum', and quoted the centre's director, Dr Michael Kelly, as follows:

> 'It is virtually impossible to deal with the volume of addicts we are now getting,' Dr Kelly says. 'We are facing a very acute situation. We can't wait for a custom-built unit to be put up. We are already choked with a motley crew of schoolchildren, hardened addicts and criminals coming in through that waiting room.'[40]

Although it had been envisaged at the time of its establishment that the Jervis Street centre would play a lead role in preventive work and in the general policy advisory area, in practice it had confined its activities almost entirely to its treatment function; this seems largely explicable in terms of the huge pressure of day-to-day clinical work which militated against the development of a reflective, analytical approach to policy issues. Not only did the Jervis Street centre fail to play a major role in alerting the Department of Health to the full significance of the rise in heroin use, but it also failed to capitalise upon its unique position in the treatment scene by securing the greatly enhanced resources it would have needed to fulfil all that was expected of it.

Given that the major increase in drug use involved heroin, the question of introducing methadone maintenance – as opposed to detoxification and drug-free rehabilitation – now had become practically relevant. The Jervis Street centre, however, did not facilitate public debate on treatment policy and, while it may have maintained some opiate users on an indefinite basis, it also retained strong links with Coolemine Therapeutic Community and generally promoted detoxification and abstinence as the treatment norm during this period. The Coolemine service expanded greatly in the early 1980s, particularly in 1983 when it acquired a new residential centre at Navan, Co. Meath, which was capable of holding up to a hundred residents. Co-operation between Jervis Street and Coolemine was close, both philosophically and practically, and between them they reinforced the most basic of the assumptions inherent in the Eastern Health Board's response to the opiate epidemic: drug addiction was largely explicable by reference to individual psychopathological characteristics; treatment was best delivered by professionals in specialist services; and the only valid outcome of treatment was total abstinence from mood-altering drugs. All of these assumptions were, to some extent at least, antipathetic towards the broad thrust of health promotion and to the specific community activities discussed in this section.

Finally, in concluding this account of the conflictual relationship between locally-based activists and statutory authorities, some reference must be made to the emergence of other forms of local community responses to drug problems in Dublin, which began in 1983 and which were frequently characterised as constituting a form of aggressive vigilantism. An umbrella body known as *Concerned Parents Against Drugs* (CPAD) sporadically provided a degree of centralised organisation for local groups who attempted to set up informal policing of their areas, and whose activities included evictions of residents judged to be drug dealers.[41] CPAD was primarily representative of residents of working-class areas, with little or no involvement of locally-based professionals, and was controversial not just for its vigilantism but because of the allegations of the authorities that it was a front for Sinn Féin. Specifically on this latter point, it was suggested that Sinn Féin was making cynical use of the heroin problem to advance its own republican political agenda. It could be argued that it was the failure of statutory bodies to collaborate and share power with more responsible and representative bodies, such as those discussed in this section, that created the conditions for the emergence of CPAD. Equally, it could be argued that the reluctance of the statutory authorities to share power was vindicated by the nature of the vigilante activities espoused by CPAD: that the Eastern Health Board, in particular, had been astute in recognising that community responses to drug users would not always be benign and that professionalism remained the best option. This is an issue which will be returned to in Chapter Seven when the question of local drug treatment services is again considered.

The Health Education Bureau and the opiate epidemic

Although it had a broad health education brief, the HEB (as discussed in Chapter Five) had been set up specifically as a result of public concern about drug problems. For the first two years of its existence it had been a rather modest affair, effectively little more than an off-shoot of the Department of Health run by a few civil servants on a small budget. During the period that Charles Haughey was Minister for Health, from July 1977 until December 1979, the fortunes of the HEB were transformed dramatically: a full-time director (Dr Harry Crawley, a consultant psychiatrist) and professional staff were appointed; a substantial budget was allocated; and a large and munificent building at Upper Mount Street in Dublin purchased as a corporate headquarters.

Despite this apparent good fortune, the environment in which the HEB was expected to operate was not entirely hospitable or uncomplicated, and it will be argued here that any analysis of the Bureau's performance must inevitably include an evaluation of its 'networking' skills or political abilities in this environment.

Paradoxically, the generosity of Charles Haughey towards the HEB may be seen as constituting a mixed blessing for the organisation. It was commonly believed and quickly confirmed that Mr Haughey was intent on using his time in the Department of Health to complete the process of political rehabilitation, necessitated by his involvement in the Arms Trial of 1970, and to position himself as successor to his Party Leader and Taoiseach, Jack Lynch. It was not uncommon then for people at this time to view Mr Haughey's commitment to health education as a cynical political exercise and, fairly or otherwise, to transfer these negative attitudes on to the HEB. The apparent wealth of the HEB also generated some resentment on the part of those already involved in health and social services who saw themselves as carrying out equally, if not more, important work in straitened circumstances. Civil servants in the Department of Health, for example, were at this time in transition from the overcrowded grandeur of the Custom House to the less salubrious environment of Hawkins House, one of Dublin's more reviled modern buildings. Statutory health and social service workers saw themselves, as perhaps they invariably do, as operating with less than adequate resources; and existing voluntary bodies, whose work had often included educational and preventive aspects, looked with a jaundiced eye at the newly acquired affluence and dominance of the HEB.

The first major initiative taken by the HEB in relation to drugs, following its transformation by Mr Haughey, was the holding of a conference on the theme of 'Education Against Addiction' in Killarney in November 1979. This conference was attended by more than three hundred delegates, from health, educational and social service backgrounds, and the speakers included national and international specialists in the addictions field. The content of the conference papers and the ensuing discussion encompassed all addictive substances – whether licit, illicit or prescribed – and the proposals which arose from the discussion referred to a wide range of public policy initiatives which, it was argued, could reduce the societal damage caused by psychoactive drug use. The final task of summarising the conference themes and recommendations fell to Jerry O'Dwyer, then a Principal Officer of the Department of Health, who referred in his summary to the 'many calls [which] were made highlighting the need for a national policy in relation to addiction'.[42] He referred specifically to two fundamental ideas which had emerged concerning:

(i)   The lack of co-ordination which was seen to exist between the many agencies who are in a position to bring resources to bear on the problem at present, and

(ii) The need to develop and implement a consistent set of attitudes and values in relation to addictions.[43]

The model of policy making implicit in these conference recommendations was the rational-comprehensive one, and the recommendations, taken as a whole, could validly be seen as health promotional. There are, however, great differences between the aspirations which delegates express at conferences and the political realities which surround their implementation. Jerry O'Dwyer, despite the clarity of his summary, must have been aware of these political difficulties, and there may have been a slight touch of mockery in his concluding wish that 'When Killarney will be but a pleasant memory for us, I hope that the bureau will publish in suitably psychedelic form the authorised version of the proceedings of the Conference and circulate it to a very wide audience'.[44]

In studying the activities of the HEB following this conference, it could be concluded that the Bureau was realistic and politically prudent in selectively pursuing conference recommendations. It did not, for example, pursue the notion of an integrated national addiction policy by developing a more active role for itself in relation to alcohol; and it seems reasonable to presume that its decision not to do so was motivated not just by a general appreciation of the difficulties inherent in bringing about a root and branch change in alcohol policy, but by a more specific and mundane desire to avoid an unseemly 'turf war' with the Irish National Council on Alcoholism.

What the HEB mainly took from this 'Education Against Addiction' conference was a renewed conviction of the validity of its position on drug education, as originally laid down by the Committee on Drug Education in 1974. This meant that it would not engage in mass media campaigns which presented the negative effects of drugs such as heroin in a sensationalist way, nor would it assist in the creation of school programmes which adopted such tactics. The Bureau was satisfied that there was no scientific justification for drug education of this kind. Not only did the research fail to show that explicit anti-drug messages delayed or prevented initiation into drug use by young people, but it also suggested that this kind of education often generated oppositional responses in its audience which ultimately could be counterproductive. The policy on drug education adopted by the HEB, therefore, was one which was low-key and non-specific; its focus was on the development of individual life-skills or decision-making skills for young people, to be achieved indirectly through training teachers, youth leaders and others who could be regarded as 'primary influencers'.

HEB policy on drug education was for all practical purposes identical to that recommended in Britain by the Advisory Council on the Misuse of Drugs in its *Prevention* report of 1984, but it is important to note that the Thatcher Government totally ignored this advice and went ahead with a large-scale advertising campaign aimed specifically at fighting heroin. In Ireland, too, it began to appear as though political leaders would prefer drug education which was more explicit, high-profile and generally propagandist, whatever the results of scientific research in this field. There emerged, therefore, an ongoing tension between the HEB's commitment to subtle educational programmes, which at least promised to do no harm, and the desires of politicians and others for a more public, full-frontal attack on heroin, symbolising society's repugnance for this drug. In a subsequent discussion of this period, Eugene Donoghue, Head of Training and Education at the Bureau, referred to the Bureau's attempts to achieve a 'fine balance between responding to public demands and conducting quality drug education'.[45]

The contrast between the measured, low-key approach of the HEB and the emerging political rhetoric of this period in the early 1980s is reflected in the words of Dr Michael Woods, Minister for Health, from a speech he made in October 1982 at the start of a seminar for school principals run by the HEB. The Minister declared dramatically that:

> The Government has declared war on drug abuse. We are determined to attack and root out this new cancer which is eating into our community. Although we were sheltered from the waves of harmful drugs which flooded Europe in the last decade, we are no longer exempt from their insidious influence.[46]

In April 1982, the Minister for Health allocated an additional £250,000 to the HEB for its drug education activities; the extra funding had not been sought and, given the implicit expectation that it would be used to conduct a more overt attack on heroin, it appeared to be regarded with some ambivalence by its recipients. Amongst those concerned with drug problems, and to some extent amongst the general public, the HEB was not viewed as an entirely credible institution, as evidenced by an *Irish Times* editorial on the subject of this extra funding, in which the wisdom of the Minister's decision was commented upon in the following way:

> Maybe he is right to increase the funding of the Health Education Bureau. Maybe their new programme will do better than those that have gone before it – although such organisations as the Coolemine Therapeutic Community (which has a proven track record in the salvage of young drug abusers) is already active in this field and is on record as being in need of further funds.[47]

This editorial comment is interesting in that it shows that, for organisations working in the drugs field, there is no necessary correlation between attention to scientific research and public credibility. The activities of the HEB, as already discussed, were carefully and conscientiously based on research findings but to the public they seemed equivocal and half-hearted. Coolemine, on the other hand, was unequivocally and whole-heartedly opposed to drugs, and to politicians and to the general public it seemed to matter not a whit that its approach to drug rehabilitation was not well supported by research evidence. The HEB did not change its policy on drug education in any way as a result of receiving this extra money from the Minister for Health, and its decision to use the money to run another international conference on drug education (which was held in the Shelbourne Hotel Dublin in November 1982) can hardly have been pleasing to the Minister and to all those who would have preferred to see it spent on something with more mass appeal.

Viewed in terms of the Ottawa Charter, the HEB's approach to drug prevention is most aptly described as 'Developing Personal Skills', an approach which is almost entirely individualistic. However, if the HEB wished to establish a popular support base for its activities, then it seemed imperative that it complement its work on individual life-skills with programmes and policies that took account of socio-economic and other environmental factors. Specifically, what would have helped the Bureau's public image and general credibility would have been the establishment of close links with the community-based groups which were attempting to deal with heroin problems in working-class areas of Dublin. Had the Bureau established such links, it would effectively have made the point that individuals do not exist in a social vacuum and that human health cannot be entirely explained in terms of personal choice. The community groups were all, with varying degrees of explicitness and coherence, developing ecological models of health which referred to their experience with heroin, and the support of the HEB might have been helpful in all kinds of ways to these groups.

There was, however, to be no real collaboration between the HEB and these community groups, a failure which can be explained in both ideological and structural/administrative terms. Ideologically, it appeared that the Bureau's view of drug problems at this time was one which was completely blind to social class and other environmental influences; as a consequence of this it concentrated exclusively on individual decision-making, ignoring social class influences and presenting all of its educational materials in a language and style which was middle class in its orientation. Dr Fergus O'Kelly, a GP who worked in the St Teresa's Gardens area of the south inner-city of Dublin and who was an active member of the Youth Development Project there, had done pioneering epidemiological work on drug problems in his practice during the early 1980s. He was, therefore, personally and professionally well placed to comment on these issues, and described his disbelief on attending an HEB seminar for doctors in 1982, at which one of the main speakers argued that drug problems were 'classless'.[48] Similarly, Dr John Bradshaw, who had carried out epidemiological research in the north inner-city of Dublin, responded critically to the Bureau's 1983 booklet *Open Your Minds to the Facts,* arguing that it was 'totally unsuited in length and tone to the parents of central Dublin and other deprived districts where drug abuse is certainly or probably rampant'.[49]

It is difficult to know why the HEB should have adopted such an individualistic stance on drug problems, given the central importance of environment in traditional public health. It is tempting, however, to conclude that it was aware of the reluctance of Government to acknowledge the link between poverty and serious drug problems, and that in opting to turn a blind eye to this link the Bureau itself was primarily motivated by a desire to avoid involvement in damaging political controversy. There was nothing unique about this determination to see drug use purely as a personal choice, and through the mid 1980s the slogan 'Just Say No' (popularised by Nancy Reagan, wife of the US President, Ronald Reagan) gained much currency internationally.

Even if it had been so minded, however, it appears that the HEB was greatly constrained by its own statutory nature when it came to working with community groups. The Bureau had been set up by the Minister for Health under the Health (Corporate Bodies) Act, 1961, a statute which allowed the Minister to establish corporate bodies to carry out health functions inappropriate to local health authorities. Both the north and south inner-city groups had sought the assistance of the HEB in their anti-drugs campaigns, but the Bureau's understanding was that it could not become involved with these groups unless permitted, if not indeed specifically requested, to do so by the statutory health authority for the area, the Eastern Health Board. In view of the on-going antagonism between the Health Board and the community groups, the Health Board demurred and so the HEB was not drawn into the picture.

It seems, in conclusion, that despite its new-found affluence the HEB played a relatively limited role in the overall health and social service response to the opiate epidemic between 1980 and 1985. Its refusal to create sensationalist and explicit advertising campaigns did not endear it to politicians who liked the high drama and symbolism of such campaigns, and its individualistic life-skills emphasis and failure to become involved with community drugs activists lost it grassroots support and credibility.

Above all perhaps, it appeared to lack the common touch when it came to networking; none of its staff developed to any great extent the communication and lobbying skills which might have served the Bureau in good stead through what was undoubtedly a difficult era. Instead, a negative perception of the HEB was allowed to develop, which included jokes about the 'lifestyle' of its personnel, referring, for example, to the grandeur of their building, the depth of their carpets and their penchant for international conferences. The Bureau moved towards a more explicit use of health promotion concepts in the mid-1980s but, despite the apparent popularity and official acceptance of such concepts, continued to be involved in public controversy. This controversy and the ultimate closure of the HEB in 1988 will be discussed in Chapter Seven.

Conclusion

The most obvious conclusion that can be drawn from the material presented in this chapter is that the various policies and institutions that had been established prior to 1980 failed to provide a speedy and effective response to the heroin problems which grew quite dramatically from this year onwards. There had been no large-scale use of opiates in Ireland prior to this time, nor had there been a culture of needle use amongst illicit drug users, and this new style of drug use brought with it a wide range of medico-social problems. Perhaps those most commented upon publicly were the risk of overdose and the drug's obvious capacity to create physical dependency, but there were also serious indirect health problems associated with needle use and needle sharing, such as hepatitis, abscesses and toxaemia. There were also behavioural problems associated with heroin use, mainly consisting of crime of an acquisitive kind aimed at raising the money necessary to sustain an illicit and expensive dependency, but prostitution as a means to 'feed a drug habit' also became more common as heroin became the primary drug of choice of illicit drug users. Such medico-social problems were of concern to Irish society as a whole but, as explained in this chapter, they particularly appeared to engulf those already deprived urban areas in which they were disproportionately prevalent.

Two bodies of which there were clear policy-making expectations – the Inter-Departmental Committee on Drug Abuse and the National Drug Advisory and Treatment Centre at Jervis Street Hospital – failed signally to meet these expectations. In the case of the former, the official explanation for its tardiness and inefficiency was couched in disingenuous bureaucratic terms: the Inter-Departmental Committee on Drug Abuse, it was suggested, did not perform well because its terms of reference were not sufficiently formal. Had it succeeded, this Inter-Departmental Committee could have been a good example of the intersectoral collaboration and co-ordination that is described under the health promotion label of 'Health Public Policy'. The evidence presented in this chapter, however, argues for an alternative explanation of why this committee was so slow to respond to the upsurge in heroin use, attributing this delay to the conservative 'territorial' instincts of Department of Health officials, who found it difficult to share administrative power or accept a policy perspective which differed from their own.

The Jervis Street centre operated solely as a clinical agency, demonstrating little interest in or aptitude for policy debate. It was telling that up to the beginning of the opiate epidemic this centre did not even compile and publish annual statistics describing its own workload. Neither, as the use of heroin increased and as its localised geographical nature became clear, did Jervis Street foster any policy debate on the merits of decentralising treatment service provision. Finally, it was significant that it largely adopted an abstinence model of treatment and rehabilitation, without any discussion of the other option, methadone maintenance, which was commonly used internationally for the treatment of heroin dependency.

The failure of these policy-making institutions meant that the kind of balanced, intersectoral debate envisaged in 'health public policy' did not occur in Ireland during this period of the opiate epidemic; as a consequence, the most visible and unequivocal policy development between 1980 and 1985 was the enactment of the Misuse of Drugs Act, 1984, which was aimed primarily at controlling the supply of illicit drugs. This legislation was, of course, broadly comparable to that being enacted internationally, but the prospect of cutting off the supply of illicit drugs through the use of criminal justice sanctions was slight; in many ways, the legislation may be considered more in terms of its symbolic importance, rather than from an instrumental perspective.

If there is any single concept which comprehensively captures the essence of the official health service response to Dublin's opiate epidemic between 1980 and 1985 it is that of *individualism*, since, both in terms of treatment service provision and health educational programmes aimed at prevention, the unit of analysis was always the individual. All of the public health or health promotional frameworks which argued that environmental factors should be considered were ignored, and a traditional biomedical model implicitly – and sometimes explicitly – underpinned all health service activities in this sphere. The 'disease' of drug dependency was seen to exist within individual sufferers and, therefore, it was in order that they should be plucked from their everyday environment and taken to a centralised treatment system, where they could be subject to the ministrations of technical experts in this condition. Health authorities seemed satisfied with this biomedical model, not so much perhaps because they were convinced of its logic or its technical efficacy but because it was familiar to them and spared them from the distasteful business of sharing power with lay people from working-class communities. For politicians, the attraction of individualism almost certainly was that it distracted public attention from the links between heroin problems and poverty; it was more comforting to conceptualise drug use in terms of the poor decision-making and defective lifestyles of individuals than to acknowledge that health is also a social product. The situation in Britain was somewhat similar, as may be gleaned from these 1984 remarks of Griffith Edwards, a psychiatrist who was recognised as one of the world's leading experts on drug problems:

> The Minister of Health will look bored if he asks us for recommendations on how to curtail the drug epidemic and we come back only with the answer that, if he does not want Brixton to go the way of Harlem he had better do something about Brixton. But if he gets the social and political job wrong, no amount of committee reports, customs officers, sniffer dogs, life sentences, consultant sessions or lecturing to school children will be able to pick up the broken pieces.[50]

These remarks apply *a fortiori* to Ireland, and Chapter Seven will look in detail at the period between 1986 and 1996, a period in which policy makers not only acknowledged that heroin use had become a permanent feature of the Irish scene but were compelled to do so in the context of the additional health risks associated with the newly-identified human immunodeficiency virus (HIV).

NOTES

1. M. Kelly, 'Misuse of a Morphine Alternative (Diconal)', *Journal of the Irish Medical Association,* 65 (1972), pp 414-415.
2. There are no Department of Health documents relating to the Inter-Departmental Committee on Drug Abuse in the public domain, and the information presented here is based on interviews with the following members of this committee: Jim Comberton, Coolemine Therapeutic Community; Joe Power, Pharmaceutical Society of Ireland; Denis Mullins, Garda Drug Squad; Martin Tansey, Principal Probation and Welfare Officer, Department of Justice; Joe O'Rourke, Assistant Secretary, Department of Health.
3. Dáil Debates (Vol. 330), Column 1384.
4. *Irish Times,* 18 November, 1981.
5. *Irish Times,* 7 December, 1981.
6. Interview with Barry Desmond, 28 November, 1988.
7. G. Dean, J. Bradshaw and P. Lavelle, *Drug Misuse in Ireland 1982-1983:*

Investigations in a North Central Dublin Area and in Galway, Sligo and Cork. (Dublin: Medico-Social Research Board, 1983).

8.   Ibid., pp 20-21.
9.   *Report of the Special Governmental Task Force on Drug Abuse, 1983,* p.1. (A leaked version of this unpublished report was procured by this writer in 1986.)
10. Ibid., p.10.
11. 'Drug Abuse and the Task Force'. (Press Release issued by the Government Information Services, 22 September, 1983.)
12. *Dáil Debates* (Vol. 351), Column 1142.
13. *Dáil Debates* (Vol. 351), Column 1146.
14. *Seanad Debates* (Vol. 104), Column 1115.
15. *Irish Council for Civil Liberties Press Release,* 22 June, 1984.
16. *Seanad Debates* (Vol. 104), Column 1119.
17. *Report of the Special Governmental Task Force on Drug Abuse,* 1983, p.18.
18. McKinsey and Co., *Towards Better Health Care Management in the Health Boards* (Vol.1). (Dublin: Department of Health, 1970), p.34.
19. Telephone interview with Michael Walsh, Programme Manager, Special Hospital Programme, Eastern Health Board, 19 December, 1988.
20. Telephone interview with Michael Walsh, 19 December, 1988.
21. Personal interview with Áine Flanagan, 29 November, 1988.
22. *Eastern Health Board Task Force on Drug Abuse.* (Unpublished report, 1983), p.1.
23. Interview with Jim Comberton, 10 October, 1988.
24. Interview with Paul Harrison, 11 November, 1988.
25. Advisory Council on the Misuse of Drugs, *Treatment and Rehabilitation.* (London: HMSO, 1982).
26. *Eastern Health Board Task Force on Drug Abuse,* cit. sup., p.3.
27. The main written sources for this section are: M.E. McCann, *Ten Years On: a history of the Ballymun Youth Action Project, a community response to drug and alcohol abuse.* (Ballymun Youth Action Project, 1991); N. O'Donohue and S. Richardson (eds), *Pure Murder: a book about drug use.* (Dublin: Women's Community Press, 1984); B. Cullen, *Community and Drugs: a case study in community conflict in the inner city of Dublin.* (M.Litt. thesis, Trinity College Dublin, 1992).

     This account also draws on previously cited research interviews with: Áine Flanagan, Eastern Health Board; Paul Harrison, Eastern Health Board; Barry Desmond, former Minister for Health. Further information was gathered from interviews with Paul Lavelle, Catholic Curate in Seán MacDermott Street in the early 1980s, and Barbara Law, social worker at the Jervis Street clinic and later at Trinity Court, Pearse Street.
28. *Submission to City Council Proposed Working Party on Drug Abuse in Dublin* (from Barry Cullen, Social Worker, Eastern Health Board Community Care Area Three, 29 October, 1981).
29. M.E. McCann, op.cit., p.11.
30. W. Martin, 'Concerned Parents Against Drugs Action Group', in N. O'Donohue and S. Richardson, op. cit., pp 71-72.
31. See G. Williams and J. Poppay, 'Lay knowledge and the privilege of experience'

in J. Gabe, D. Kelleher and G. Williams (eds), *Challenging Medicine*. (London: Routledge, 1994), pp 118-134.

32.   B. Cullen, op.cit., p.63.

33.   See, for instance, P. Malone, 'Community Action in the North Inner City, in N. O'Donohue and S. Richardson, op.cit., pp 75-81.

34.   Letter from Mary Aylward, Department of Health, to Tom Harty, Eastern Health Board (dated 25 May, 1982) describing a meeting between representatives from the Seán MacDermott Street parish and the Minister for Health.

35.   *Irish Times,* 4 February, 1985.

36.   See M.E. McCann, op. cit.

37.   World Health Organisation, *Targets for Health for All.* (Copenhagen: WHO Regional Office for Europe, 1985). It is worth noting that this WHO publication had considerable currency in Irish health policy circles and was an influence on two policy documents – *Health: The Wider Dimensions* (1986) and *Promoting Health Through Public Policy* (1987).

38.   This account is based on numerous dealings which this writer had with Áine Flanagan in relation to alcohol and drug services between 1977 and 1991, and on a research interview with her on 28 November, 1988.

39.   In his research interview with this writer, Paul Harrison commented humorously that, in terms of the Health Board culture of this period, 'planning was for sissies'; and the former Minister for Health, Barry Desmond, was emphatic that any attempt to discuss drug policy issues with Fred Donohue (Programme Manager for Community Care at this time) quickly degenerated into farce as Mr Donohue overwhelmed him with personal anecdotes.

40.   *Irish Times*, 23 November, 1983.

41.   For a succinct analyis of the origins of CPAD in the broader context of community work in Ireland see B. Cullen, 'Community Action in the Eighties: A Case Study' in *Community Work in Ireland: Trends in the 80s, Options for the 90s.* (Dublin: Combat Poverty Agency, 1990), pp 271-294.
       For a sympathetic sociological view of CPAD as an informal policing system see D. Bennett, 'Are They Always Right? Investigation and proof in a citizen anti-heroin movement' in M. Tomlinson, T. Varley and C. McCullagh (eds), *Whose Law and Order? Aspects of crime and social control in Irish society.* (Sociological Association of Ireland, 1988), pp 21-40.

42.   J. O'Dwyer, 'Conference Report and Recommendations' in *Education Against Addiction.* (Dublin: Health Education Bureau, no date), p.90.

43.   Ibid., p.90.

44.   Ibid., p.93.

45.   E. Donoghue, 'Drug Education: Approaches in Ireland'. *Paper read at International Symposium on the Health-Promoting School at Peebles, Scotland, 11-17 May , 1986,* p.10.

46.   *Press Release issued by the Government Information Services on behalf of the Department of Health, 5 October, 1982.*

47.   *Irish Times, 27 April, 1982.*

48.   Cited in B. Cullen, 1992, cit. sup., p.53.

49.   *Irish Times, 25 July, 1983.*

50.   G. Edwards, 'Addiction: A Challenge to Society', *New Society* (October 25, 1984), p.135.

7

Coping with 'The Virus' 1986-1996: Irish Drug Policy in the Age of HIV

Introduction

The period of the 'opiate epidemic', which was the subject of Chapter Six, was for Irish drug policy makers a difficult one. The apparent consensus amongst all sectors of Government, and amongst the general population, on the evils of illicit drug use neither prevented the emergence of a serious heroin problem nor did it lead automatically to the formulation and implementation of clear and effective policy in this area. On the contrary, it can fairly be said that the sudden upsurge in heroin use from 1979 onwards appeared to take the authorities by surprise and that they struggled to come to terms with the complexities of this new situation. Policy making during the period 1986-1996, which is the subject of the present chapter, was to be an even more fraught affair. Not only did Irish policy makers have to cope with all of the unresolved issues and dilemmas from the earlier period, but they were now compelled to review the most basic tenets of conventional drug policy in the light of the new public health crisis created by the human immunodeficiency virus (HIV) and its associated acquired immune deficiency syndrome (AIDS).

This chapter will analyse the drug policy response in the era of what Dublin drug users tended to refer to simply as 'the virus'. Bearing in mind the radically changed policy climate engendered by HIV/AIDS, the focus here will again be on the way in which policy makers devised individualistic and environmental strategies, and on the way in which they handled the balance between these strategies. In addition to this, the policy process itself will be considered with a view to seeing which of the policy models used throughout this book corresponds most closely to the policy process during this period.

HIV/AIDS and their impact on drug policy

Prior to the advent of HIV/AIDS, it could be said that Irish drug policy was a seamless garment in which all sectors of government were agreed on the absolute evil of illicit drugs and on the necessity to work collaboratively for the attainment of a drug-free society. In *Health: The Wider Dimensions,* a consultative document on health promotion published by the Department of Health in 1986, there was a brief statement to the effect that: 'In Ireland the problem of drug abuse provides a good example of intersectoral collaboration working successfully in practice'.[1] This statement was by way of contrast with an immediately preceding discussion of the difficulties involved in fostering an intersectoral response to alcohol problems in Ireland. Sociologists have tended to view *health risk* as a social construct rather than as solely, or even primarily, the product of objective and value-free research; what this means is that societal decisions about what are deemed to be hazards or dangers to human health are arrived at through social, cultural and political processes rather than always flowing rationally and directly from scientific research.

Applying this notion of health risk to what has been presented thus far in this book, it could be said that Irish society has demonstrated a marked reluctance to acknowledge alcohol consumption as an essentially risky activity – despite the best efforts of public health activists who argued for such a construction. On the other hand, it could be said that discourse on the health risks of illicit drug use was exaggerated, since there was virtually no voice to argue for a more subtle or discriminating analysis of how these drugs had an adverse impact on human health. It will be argued in this chapter, however, that in common with other countries, Ireland was compelled to question this absolutist or fundamentalist rejection of drugs, once the connection between HIV transmission and needle sharing between intravenous drug users began to become clear in the mid-1980s. When drug use and HIV infection were viewed in relative public health terms, it began to seem as though drug use was the lesser of two evils; therefore newer approaches to drug policy, reflecting this conclusion, began to emerge. This abandonment of the absolutist rhetoric of the War on Drugs effectively constituted a rending of the previously seamless garment of Irish drug policy: the criminal justice system might continue to enforce prohibitionist laws, and the educational system might continue to exhort Irish young people to remain drug-free, but there could be no gainsaying the fact that, in response to the crisis of HIV/AIDS, Irish health policy was moving towards a position in which total abstinence was no longer seen as the only acceptable treatment outcome for illicit drug users.

From a policy perspective, the introduction of HIV prevention measures in Ireland was unusually complex. As would later become clear, the task of ensuring that blood and blood products were uncontaminated was far from simple, but it could at least be said that this was a task which was essentially technical and which was not complicated by moral debate.

When the focus is switched to HIV prevention amongst gay men and intravenous drug users, it becomes instantly clear that the policy process is greatly complicated by moral debate, because the behaviours involved were illegal and commonly regarded as morally reprehensible.[2] From the mid-1980s onwards, the Department of Health – with the technical assistance of the Virus Reference Laboratory at University College Dublin – monitored the incidence of HIV infection in Ireland, and this epidemiological research was intended to be used as a basis for planning preventive strategies.

Table 9: Antibody positive test results in selected samples of at risk groups in Ireland (November, 1985)

At Risk Group	No. Tested	% Positive
Haemophiliacs	256	33
Intravenous Drug Abusers	240	30
Homosexuals	347	9

Source: Department of Health, 1986

Preliminary HIV testing, as can be seen from Table 9, revealed that haemophiliacs had indeed been badly affected by contaminated blood products used in the treatment of their illness; however, it also confirmed that gay men and intravenous drug users constituted important 'at risk' groups for whom the construction of prevention strategies was likely to be a complex and ongoing process. Prevention campaigns could, of course, have been confined to simple admonitions to these latter groups to stay within the law and desist from illicit sexual and drug use behaviours, which now carried an additional risk of exposure to HIV. Such preventive tactics were generally deemed futile, however, and policy makers in Ireland, as elsewhere, were led to a consideration of more pragmatic measures to deal with this major public health problem. What gave further impetus to this switch towards pragmatism was the conclusion on the part of public health authorities that HIV/AIDS was unlikely to be confined to these 'deviant' sub-groups, but that these groups might act as a bridge for the transmission of HIV into the general population. Such transmission could occur, for instance, when drug users had sexual contacts with non-drug users, or when bisexual men became infected through homosexual contacts and then went on to infect their women partners.

Despite the fact that male homosexual behaviour was still illegal, the Health Education Bureau gave funding to a voluntary body known as the

Gay Health Action group, which led to the production of the state's first information leaflets on AIDS, in 1985 and 1988. These leaflets did not advocate sexual abstinence for gay people but instead recommended what came to be known as 'safer sex' practices – such as non-penetrative sex or the use of condoms – which minimised the risk of HIV transmission. To put these Gay Health Action activities in context, it should be pointed out that the laws against male homosexual activity were by this time rarely enforced and that a legal and political campaign for the decriminalisation of male homosexuality was well under way.

There was, however, absolutely no suggestion from any quarter that the ideological basis of Irish drug policy and legislation was in need of revision. The legislation was of recent origin and strictly enforced, and, as discussed in Chapter Six, many Irish politicians tended to the view that their public pronouncements on drug issues should be unequivocally prohibitionist. Furthermore, illicit drug users were generally regarded as a disparate and disorganised collection of individuals, primarily to be categorised in pathological terms, rather than viewed as a coherent lobby group like the 'gay community'. Nonetheless, for public health policy in Ireland an obvious dilemma had arisen: the prevention of HIV transmission had become imperative, but it was impossible to see how effective preventive measures could be introduced amongst intravenous drug users without apparently undermining the ideological commitment to a drug-free society as epitomised in the Misuse of Drugs Acts. Just as HIV prevention in the gay community revolved around safer sex rather than sexual abstinence, so too was it now mooted that amongst drug users it might consist of safer drug use rather than solely being confined to the traditional therapeutic goal of total abstinence. The phrase most commonly used to describe this emerging public health approach to drug use was 'harm reduction', and its meaning and implications will now be discussed in some detail.

Harm reduction

It could be argued that traditional drug treatment and rehabilitation programmes which aim to make their clients drug free merit the title *harm reduction*; such programmes are, after all, concerned with reducing drug-related harm and do so in what is the most obvious way, which is to assist drug users to become and remain drug free. In the context of the public health crisis associated with HIV, however, harm reduction is invariably understood as referring to strategies which are aimed at reducing drug-related harm where drug users are either unwilling or unable to stop using drugs. The concept of harm reduction, when understood in this context, incorporated some strategies, such as methadone maintenance, which were not new, and some others, such as needle exchange schemes, which were devised specifically in response to HIV.[3]

While proponents of harm reduction tended to the view that such strategies were pragmatic responses, which were justified in the era of HIV/AIDS and were necessitated by the obvious failure of abstinence approaches, opposition to harm reduction was predictable. Essentially, the emergence and articulation of a harm reduction philosophy involved a fundamental reconstruction of drug-related health risk in a way which was ideologically undermining of the traditional prohibitionist position. For example, in relation to heroin use, it was now being acknowledged that it was not heroin use *per se* which constituted the major health risk (although there were overdose risks associated with heroin), but rather the practice of administering the drug intravenously with non-sterile injecting equipment. This acknowledgement led logically to a consideration of a number of HIV prevention strategies for heroin users. Harm reduction and abstinence are not necessarily dichotomous categories, and in practice many professionals would start by suggesting to their heroin-using clients that they should detoxify and remain abstinent. Where clients were unable or unwilling to pursue the abstinence option, however, there were now several other harm reduction options which could be explored, including the following:

- the replacement of street heroin by a prescribed substitute drug, such as methadone, which is usually taken orally
- the use of heroin through smoking rather than by injection
- intravenous use by means of sterile, non-shared injecting equipment – made available through needle exchange schemes
- intravenous use by means of shared equipment, where the user is given advice and assistance in the art of sterilising previously used needles and syringes.

Individually and collectively these harm reduction options represented a new style of risk construction in terms of the health implications of illicit drug use; what they acknowledged explicitly was that it was not drug use *per se* which constituted the sole or even the major risk to human health and that it should logically be possible to foster 'healthy' drug use, just as it was logically possible, for example, to foster 'sensible drinking'.

If the various harm reduction strategies are considered in more depth, it becomes clear that they differ from the traditional abstinence approach not just in that they tolerate continuing drug use, but also in that they involve a radical reconceptualisation of drug users. Prior to the advent of HIV the dominant conceptualisation of illicit drug users had been grounded in ideas of pathology. Drug use was regarded as a self-evidently pathological and deviant activity; individual drug users were assumed to demonstrate high levels of individual psychopathology; and insofar as drug users were perceived to exist within their own sub-culture this too tended to be seen in sociopathological terms. The emergence of treatment and rehabilitation services for illicit drug users in Ireland, as discussed in Chapters Five and Six, had been completely predicated upon such pathological conceptualisations of drug users. Implicit in the harm reduction approach to drug treatment services, however, was a very different view of illicit drug users, one which was more positive and respectful.

Harm reduction philosophy reframed illicit drug use as a phenomenon which was just as intelligible as alcohol consumption, and the decision of illicit drug users to seek gratification in this way was no longer regarded as inherently irrational or pathological. Furthermore, it came to be accepted that the process of maximising drug-related pleasure while minimising risk was just as amenable to health promotion interventions as any other aspect of lifestyle. Most important of all perhaps, was the related acceptance of the view that health care professionals could no longer assume a position of moral and cognitive superiority in their dealings with illicit drug users. Instead, in the new dispensation, it was argued in classic health promotional terms that professionals should respect and learn from the knowledge and wisdom of drug users, who, it was argued, knew more about drug use than anybody else. It was suggested, for instance, that current drug users could play a valuable role in health promotion as *peer workers* in their own drug-using communities. In a 1989 paper in which he attempted to summarise the shift towards harm reduction in the British treatment scene, Griffith Edwards suggested that:

> The central change is perhaps that the balance of power between treatment agency and person treated has been sharply re-adjusted. Agencies have less capacity than previously to demand, challenge, set contracts or exclude from treatment, while patients or clients are now likely to secure treatment (including prescribed opiates) much more on their own terms.[4]

Also implicit in this more positive and respectful vision of drug users was a conviction that services should be structured in such a way as to maximise their acceptability and accessibility to potential consumers; centralised services (such as those which had been set up in Dublin) to which drug users were expected to come as supplicants were no longer viewed as appropriate, and it came to be expected that services would be localised and that *outreach* systems would be set in place to make contact with hitherto untreated drug users.[5]

Given the vehemence of international condemnations of illicit drugs and the uncompromising nature of the rhetoric of the War on Drugs, it was obvious that the introduction of harm reduction policies would be difficult and contentious everywhere. Ideologically, harm reduction represented a softening of the anti-drugs stance which had previously been unchallenged; to those who remained fully committed to the prohibitionist stance, harm reduction was an unacceptable compromise which looked suspiciously like the first steps towards decriminalisation, if not full legalisation, of previously prohibited substances. From a comparative perspective, one could predict that some countries would have less difficulty than others in introducing harm reduction, depending not just on how particular countries had framed their own drug policy but also on their wider political cultures. For instance, in view of its previous history of the so-called 'British system' (which could logically be regarded as an early experiment with harm reduction), it could be predicted that Britain would experience far less problems in introducing harm reduction than would the USA, which had historically given a dominant role to the criminal justice system and allowed little or no discretion to medical practitioners. Similarly it seemed clear that the Netherlands – with a political culture which was generally characterised by pragmatism – had already been introducing a harm reduction policy (although without naming it as such) for ten years prior to the identification of HIV.[6]

The total reorientation of health services for drug users which was implicit in harm reduction was obviously likely to prove difficult for Irish policy makers. Dublin services had been entirely centralised, insistent on abstinence as the only acceptable treatment goal and unwilling to share power with local community groups. It was hard to see how these services could be easily decentralised, how methadone maintenance or needle and syringe exchange schemes could be widely introduced, and how power could be shared with drug users in outreach and peer-led service initiatives.

Even if political leaders in Ireland felt personally inclined to advocate the introduction of harm reduction strategies – and it has to be said that during the mid-1980s there was little evidence of such inclination – the political climate at this time could hardly have been less favourable to such a liberal-seeming enterprise. The success of conservative religious groups in the 1983 'pro-life' Constitutional Referendum and in the 1986 Constitutional Referendum on divorce had created unprecedented social divisions and must surely have convinced politicians that this was not an opportune time for the introduction of what would generally be seen as liberalised drug policies. The capacity of these 'faith-based' groupings to have a political impact will now be looked at specifically in relation to the controversy which arose concerning the Health Education Bureau's lifeskills programme, following which the remainder of this chapter will look in detail at how drug-treatment systems responded to the HIV/AIDS issue.

The Health Education Bureau and the lifeskills controversy

As indicated in Chapter Six, the HEB had resolutely ignored the structural and environmental aspects of Dublin's drug problems, opting instead for an exclusive focus on individual decision-making insofar as its preventive activities in this sphere were concerned. It might, therefore, have expected to avoid being drawn into political controversy but this was not to be. The programme of lifeskills education devised by the HEB, and for which training was provided to teachers and other youth workers, was quintessentially health promotional in its non-authoritarian or partnership approach to this task. Students were not instructed to make particular behavioural choices, such as saying no to drugs; instead, they were encouraged in a non-directive way to explore the scientific data on the relevant health risks, to consider the nature of peer pressure and other pressures to make certain choices, and to clarify their value systems in relation to their lifestyle options.[7]

From the mid-1980s, however, a number of conservative Roman Catholic groupings started to develop a coherent, sustained and public critique of lifeskills programmes generally and of the HEB in particular. These critics based their objections on their belief in objective moral truth and on what they saw as the related duty of teachers to instruct their charges in this morality. The initial criticisms came from lay members of the Catholic Church[8] who argued that lifeskills education was secular, humanist and fundamentally antithetical to traditional Christian methods of religious and moral education. Later, some of the more conservative members of the Roman Catholic Hierarchy – notably Dr Kevin McNamara, Archbishop of Dublin, and Dr Jeremiah Newman, Bishop of Limerick added their voice to this criticism.[9] The HEB seemed taken aback at this attack on its approach to health education, unhappy at the ensuing public controversy, and unsure as to how to respond. In September 1987, the Minister for Health announced the closure of the HEB and its replacement by a body to be called the *Health Promotion Unit* within his own department. The closure of the HEB was certainly not brought about solely by ideological conflict about lifeskills, but as one of its sternest critics, Doris Manly, wrote:

> Why did the government axe the HEB? I don't know. Did our criticism play much of a part in the decision? Again, I don't know. I think it reasonable to assume that it may have played some part. But how large a one it's impossible even to speculate. The one safe conclusion, I suppose, is that our criticism didn't do the HEB any good.[10]

It is instructive to compare the lot of the HEB with that of the National Social Services Board (NSSB), the closure of which was announced at about the same time as that of the HEB. While the HEB appeared to accept its fate stoically, the NSSB mounted a vigorous and successful campaign, drawing on its national network of voluntary community information workers, to have this decision rescinded. Again, this demonstrated the failure of the HEB to develop a community base.

In the broader context of HIV/AIDS, the real significance of this debacle about the morality of lifeskills was that it signalled that the introduction of harm reduction strategies into the drug treatment system had the potential to arouse similar controversy. Despite the public health risks associated with a continuance of abstinence models of treatment, the Department of Health could not assume that there would be automatic acceptance of methadone maintenance, needle exchange or free condom distribution.

Making the transition to harm reduction

The new National Co-ordinating Committee on Drug Abuse, which had been recommended in 1983, was established by the Minister for Health in March 1985 with the following formal terms of reference:

(i)   to advise the Government on general issues relating to the prevention and treatment of drug abuse
(ii)   to monitor the effectiveness and efficiency of measures in force to prevent and treat drug abuse
(iii)   to facilitate communication between the various agencies involved in the prevention and treatment of drug abuse
(iv)   to submit a report to the Minister for Health on an annual basis.

This committee was not established on a statutory basis, but presumably the requirement that it submit an annual report to the Minister was seen as offering a reasonable prospect that it would survive as an active standing committee, unlike its predecessor.

The committee's chair was a politician, Fergus O'Brien, who was at this time Minister of State at the Department of the Environment and who, by virtue of his previous experience as chair of the Special Governmental Task Force on Drug Abuse during 1982 and 1983, seemed highly suited to this task. The committee itself was made up of a mix of civil servants, healthcare professionals, senior members of the Garda Síochána, representatives of the voluntary and community sector, and some others. Once again, however, the committee was based in the Department of Health and was reliant for research, administrative and secretarial support on the staff of that department. Its *First Annual Report* was published in

June 1986, fifteen months after its inaugural meeting, and it was indicated in this report that the committee had met on eight occasions during this initial fifteen-month period.[11] This could be regarded as an acceptably frequent record of meetings, but there were already ominous signs that the committee was sliding into the pattern of its predecessor of the 1970s.

From a procedural perspective, the most significant change in the makeup of the committee was the resignation during this period of its chairperson, Fergus O'Brien, and his replacement by Liam Flanagan, Secretary of the Department of Health. The reason cited for this change was Mr O'Brien's heavy workload at this time, but indeed it seemed predictable that such a busy politician – dividing his time between the Oireachtas, his departmental responsibilities in the Department of the Environment and his constituency work – would not be the ideal person to chair a committee such as this. The fact that the chairperson was now a senior civil servant from the Department of Health meant that the new committee had effectively reverted to the position of the discredited Inter-Departmental Committee of the 1970s, with control of the agenda and of the frequency of meetings once more back in the hands of departmental officials.

Equally importantly, a reading of the contents of the committee's first report would suggest that it was working in a relatively superficial administrative way, side-stepping policy issues and dilemmas and confining itself to cursory and uncritical comment on the topics it had discussed. For instance, its paragraph on lifeskills consisted of brief references to the development of lifeskills programmes in the Eastern and the North-Western Health Board areas, and to the necessity for extending these programmes to the country as a whole. It referred neither to the results of evaluative research on these programmes (which at best were only moderately encouraging) nor to the political controversy over lifeskills which was brewing at this time.

It is, however, in relation to HIV/AIDS that the reluctance of the National Co-ordinating Committee on Drug Abuse to engage in critical policy debate becomes most pointed. The 1986 report contained just one page of desultory comment on this subject, with no reference to harm reduction or to the policy dilemmas inherent in responding to the transmission of HIV amongst intravenous heroin users. An equivalent amount of space was given in the report to an uncritical recording of the views expressed to the committee by a visiting American, Ms Carla Lowe of the *Californians for Drug-Free Youth,* a parents' anti-drugs organisation. Amongst these views were Ms Lowe's stated conviction that 'children from all backgrounds were involved' in drug abuse, and that cannabis 'is possibly the most dangerous of all drugs'.[12]

Following the publication of this 1986 report, the National Co-ordinating Committee on Drug Abuse went into a period of drift, meeting rarely and never publishing another annual report. In 1989 the committee was 're-constituted', which meant that almost all those nominally members of it were replaced, largely by civil servants, and this re-constituted committee went on to produce a policy document, the *Government Strategy to Prevent Drug Misuse* in 1991. This 1991 report will be discussed later in the chapter, but first it seems important to comment upon the failure of yet another policy-making body to function as intended.

The most obvious interpretation of the failure of this committee to function in accordance with its formal terms of reference again involves the Department of Health's distaste for power-sharing or for adopting a social networks approach to policy making. The committee had no statutory existence and, once the position of chair was abandoned by its political holder, power effectively reverted to the civil service. As already indicated, the committee reflected a wide – and to some extent conflicting – range of interests and views; it appears as though the civil servants were loath to act as mediators or network builders, opting instead to retain power for themselves by simply not calling meetings.[13] It is interesting for comparative purposes to note that in Britain the Advisory Council on the Misuse of Drugs, which as a statutory body enjoyed a considerable amount of autonomy, debated the implications of HIV/AIDS for drugs policy more explicitly and more overtly. It published a number of reports on this topic, the first of which recommended the adoption of harm reduction strategies based on the much-quoted premise that 'The spread of HIV is a greater danger to individual and public health than drug misuse'.[14]

Given the failure of the National Co-ordinating Committee to debate harm reduction issues, the likelihood of any formal debate of the topic seemed slight. However, in early 1988, Seanad Éireann had a debate on AIDS to which the Minister for Health, Dr Rory O'Hanlon, and his Minister of State, Terry Leydon contributed. Senators David Norris and Joe O'Toole had arranged briefings on HIV/AIDS for their colleagues immediately prior to the debate and, whether because of these briefings by experts in this area or because of a long-term interest in the subject, the contributions seemed extremely well informed. Almost all of the speakers took the view that HIV constituted such a threat to public health that it warranted a revision of the previous tradition of abstinence as the sole legitimate model for drug treatment and rehabilitation services. Furthermore, Senators who took this view were aware of the moral dilemmas which this entailed but felt that it was a policy nettle which had to be grasped. For instance, Dr John O'Connell spoke as follows:

> This is very disturbing. It is important to have energetic preventive measures targeted at this high risk group. It would do much to ensure that the epidemic here is controlled. I can understand the dilemma of the Minister and his Department. It is a very serious thing as to whether they should conspire in illegal acts, but free needle provision and methadone maintenance must be seriously considered by the Department ... Here the objections are raised. If you are going to provide needles, like methadone maintenance, it looks very like collusion with illegal activity, but with AIDS we are facing a problem of such enormity, such potential disaster for the human race that collusion is amply justified. I urge urgently [sic] on the Minister to make a decision on it as fast as possible.[15]

By and large, his colleagues agreed with Dr O'Connell, and in various ways expressed support for a radical rethink of policy approaches to drug users. Senator Nuala Fennell, for example, was just one speaker to refer to the Dutch idea of having a 'junkies union' in which the knowledge and skills of drug users could be harnessed in a health promotional way – 'It may be an outrageous idea, but is well worth looking at'.[16]

The ghost at this harm-reduction feast was Senator Don Lydon, a Fianna Fáil Senator, who argued trenchantly that communal moral standards must be maintained whatever the gravity of the HIV/AIDS situation. The flavour of Senator Lydon's contribution may be gauged from his assertion that: 'The whole population is not at risk. Drug addicts and promiscuous people are at risk. Sodomites are certainly at risk'.[17]

The most important speech of all in this debate, perhaps, was that of the Minister, Dr O'Hanlon. He had spoken first and so was uninfluenced by any of the subsequent speeches, but obviously his views were a disappointment to those who later argued for harm reduction. The Minister's speech had all the appearances of a carefully-drafted civil service text: it was orderly and factually detailed, yet it managed to avoid all reference to the policy dilemmas which this situation created for a Minister for Health. He referred to just one policy innovation in the drugs treatment system in Dublin, namely the establishment of an outreach programme for drug users within the Eastern Health Board, but this was a brief reference which did not review the wider treatment service systems and their appropriateness for the new challenges posed by HIV. Towards the end of his speech he made the following brief reference to harm reduction:

> We are also monitoring what is happening in other countries in relation to the availability of free needles for drug abusers and also the use of methadone. To date we are not satisfied that we should go in that direction but we are monitoring the situation very closely and when we are satisfied we will make a decision in whatever way we think is best.[18]

By comparison with most of the other contributions to this debate in Seanad Éireann (and no single debate of a comparable nature took place in Dáil Éireann), the Minister's speech was remarkably stilted and cautious, and it might reasonably be inferred from it that he had decided that harm reduction was unacceptable to the Irish public and that even to debate it was unwise.

The reality, however, was more complex than this, because even at the time of this debate in Seanad Éireann harm-reduction strategies were already being introduced; what was happening was that, without formal debate or public announcement of policy change, methadone maintenance was now being used more commonly in the National Drug Advisory and Treatment Centre at Jervis Street Hospital. Furthermore, the Eastern Health Board was planning a major expansion of its own direct services for drug users, and the new EHB services – which were to be based in an *AIDS Resource Centre* at the old Baggot Street Hospital – were to include not just methadone maintenance but also needle exchange. It could perhaps be argued that this introduction of harm-reduction strategies without public debate or formal policy announcement was not all that unusual, but that it corresponded to a common pattern of incremental policy change. What was remarkable was that such a policy shift – however incrementally it may have been introduced – was taking place at the same time as the Minister for Health was publicly indicating that he did not support such a revision of traditional policy. While those whose day-to-day work involved them in contact with drug issues may have been aware of this contradiction, it did not impinge itself forcibly on to public consciousness or give rise to comment. An interesting exception was the reporting by the *Irish Times* of a speech by Dr O'Hanlon in November 1988, at the opening of the *National Drug Treatment Centre* – a new unit necessitated by the closure of Jervis Street Hospital. The Minister's speech was reported in the following terms:

> There is insufficient evidence to support the introduction of free condoms or needle exchange for drug abusers, the Minister for Health, Dr O'Hanlon, said at the opening of a major new drugs treatment unit in Dublin yesterday ... Dr O'Hanlon's remarks seem to cut across those made by the head of the Government's AIDS programme, Dr James Walsh, who earlier in the day had come out in favour of free condoms and needles for drug abusers.[19]

This quote is valuable both as an indication of how paradoxical this policy situation could appear when it was explicitly adverted to, and as confirmation of the way in which public health concerns about AIDS were now driving drug policy in Ireland.

It would be wrong to suppose that Ireland was uniquely affected by this policy dilemma, in which the health sector appeared to be breaking ranks with the criminal justice approach to working for a drug-free society. Nutbeam, Blakey and Pates (1991), in an international review of the issues involved in promoting health amongst injecting drug users, argued that:

> Making such a shift in policy has been a difficult task in many countries. Where it has happened, it has often occurred by default and without overt political support ... A better understanding of the issues and seriousness of the public health problem has led to more rational and pragmatic policy responses, based on well presented public health arguments. However, these experiences indicate how important it is not to underestimate the difficulties and dilemmas facing policy makers who are being urged to overturn established public policy, and to run counter to public opinion.[20]

Bearing in mind, therefore, that the introduction of harm reduction strategies was a contentious business in many countries, the next section will look in further detail at the implementation of these practices in Ireland. It will be argued that this incremental introduction of harm reduction, without formal debate or public announcement – which of course flies in the face of conventional ideas about policy transparency – can be seen as having both positive and negative consequences from a health promotional perspective.

The *pros* and *cons* of covert harm reduction

Throughout the period covered in this chapter (1986-1996) harm-reduction services and facilities were introduced in the covert, incremental way already described, and it was only towards the end of this period that this policy change began to be overtly discussed or explicitly acknowledged. Because change was introduced into the Dublin drug treatment system in this stealthy fashion it is not easy to be entirely accurate about when specific developments took place, but some of the more important events and initiatives are set out chronologically in Table 10.

*Table 10: Introduction of harm-reduction practices into the Dublin drug treatment
system*

1987	Increased availability of methadone maintenance at the National Drug Treatment Centre
1989	Establishment by Eastern Health Board of AIDS Resource Centre, offering needle exchange, methadone maintenance and outreach work
1991-1993	Establishment of localised 'satellite' clinics by Eastern Health Board, again offering needle exchange and methadone maintenance
1996	Introduction of mobile clinic/methadone bus

From the perspective of those concerned about promoting health amongst
Dublin's injecting drug users, the main advantage of this low-key and
incremental policy change was that it confused opponents of harm
reduction and avoided the emergence of public controversy such as that
which had bedevilled the Health Education Bureau's lifeskills programme.
The ambiguity surrounding this policy shift meant that there was no
clearly identifiable target for those ideologically opposed to harm
reduction, and this undoubtedly contributed to the fact that no sustained
and coherent campaign for a return to 'abstinence only' policies emerged
over the course of this decade.

It should be noted, however, that opposition to such practices as needle
exchange and methadone maintenance was expressed sporadically, usually
emanating from groups committed to the idea of abstinence as the only
legitimate therapeutic goal for drug users as well as to the wider aspiration
to a drug-free society. One of the key players in the voluntary drug sector
in Dublin, the Coolemine Therapeutic Community, had its origins in
American models of rehabilitation which were axiomatically committed to
abstinence. As described in Chapters Five and Six, the Coolemine
programme, from the time of its establishment in 1973, had been
reasonably well funded from statutory sources and generally treated with
deference by other stakeholders in the drug problems arena. In the early
1980s, before the identification of HIV, Jim Comberton, Executive
Chairman of the Coolemine service had circulated in photocopy form a
paper entitled 'The Self-fulfilling Prophesy [sic] of Physeptone
Maintenance (1)'. This pre-emptive strike against those who might lobby
for the introduction of methadone maintenance in Ireland was written in
uncompromising, polemical language, concluding:

There have been no Government proposals or official speculation about the introduction of Physeptone Maintenance in the Republic of Ireland, and we have no reason to expect proposals in this direction. Our concern, drawing on the disastrous experience of other countries, is that we be ready to challenge the use of Physeptone Maintenance and make its rejection a matter of public policy.[21]

Jim Comberton's readiness to challenge *proposals* for the introduction of methadone maintenance was obviously frustrated by the fact that no such proposals were ever made. Instead, the practice was introduced discreetly into the healthcare system, making it difficult for its opponents to know when it had started, how widespread it was, or even whether it was being done with Governmental approval.

A similar, but more lengthy document, was circulated by Jim Comberton in 1990, entitled 'Ireland's Young People Have a Right to a Drug-Free Life'. Again, what was most interesting about this 1990 paper was the sense that its author, while realising that the harm-reduction policy to which he was opposed was 'in the air', was confused as to what precisely was happening. The content of the paper was primarily aimed at demonstrating that methadone maintenance and needle exchange were discredited British and Dutch social control policies – rather than therapeutic initiatives – and also that such policies were immoral. On the question of the morality of harm reduction, there was an interesting reference (perhaps a tilt at some of the priests who were now involved in harm reduction) back to the 'Very high aspirations and principles [which] were voiced during the Right to Life controversy', and it was concluded that:

It is surely unacceptable that any Catholic organisation would be involved in getting drugs for addicts. In fact, His Holiness, Pope John Paul has been very vehement on this issue, and the rights of addicts, and has stated that 'you can't cure drug addicts with drugs'.[22]

However, on the question of what practical changes in service provision had occurred, Comberton was apparently on less sure ground. There was a reference to the Eastern Health Board's AIDS Resource Centre early in this 1990 paper, which Comberton interpreted as evidence that 'the Eastern Health Board has been pressured into introducing a centre for the distribution of needles and Methadone'. Towards the end of the paper, however, he suggested that:

We must be appreciative of the fact that to date neither the Irish Department of Justice or [sic] the Department of Health have pursued social control, or social engineering, policies in relation to drug addicts. There is now, however, pressure on the Department of Health to adopt the UK approach.[23]

This paper concludes by discussing the pressure on the Minister for Health to bow to harm-reduction advocates, a pressure which Comberton urges him to resist because 'We cannot allow our ethical standards to be eroded or set aside'.[24]

Although Coolemine Therapeutic Community continued to espouse abstinence policies, it never mounted a high-profile or sustained public attack on harm-reduction policy, and as the 1990s progressed its public opposition to harm reduction was confined to occasional feature articles or the letters' columns in newspapers.

There were other professionals or lobbyists whose opposition to harm reduction also received occasional publicity. Amongst these was Gráinne Kenny, who was originally a member of Community Action on Drugs (CAD), an Irish organisation, and who then went on to represent Ireland in an international organisation, Europe Against Drugs (EURAD), which was vehemently opposed to harm reduction. And finally, as an example of the opposition to harm reduction which surfaced periodically amongst healthcare professionals, reference will be made here to the discussion which took place on this topic at the AGM of the Irish Medical Organisation (IMO) in October 1989. In view of the perceived gravity of the HIV/AIDS situation, it was decided that the IMO was 'to push for the introduction without delay of comprehensive methadone maintenance and needle exchange programmes and for educational publicity aimed towards at-risk groups'. The debate on this issue was by no means characterised by unanimity, however, and it was reported that one contributor argued that:

> [I]t was time we spoke about the vast majority of people who are not perverts or addicts but who were paying their taxes and rearing their children and could not get treatment. There were people who needed hip replacements, immobile by day, sleepless by night, who might have to wait three years for their operation. These were honest to God people in our community who had to do without because of the allocation to these people.[25]

It appears however as though opponents of harm reduction were outmanoeuvred by this tactic of implementing new policy without first going through the conventional preliminaries of debate and public announcement. If the National Co-ordinating Committee on Drug Abuse had debated the introduction of harm reduction, the process would almost certainly have been slow and acrimonious, and might have given rise to general public controversy on the morality of this policy change. Instead, as was the case with the earlier Inter-Departmental Committee during the 1970s, the National Co-ordinating Committee was consigned to limbo – rarely meeting and doing no real work – while departmental officials effectively controlled policy events in this sphere. What was different during the latter half of the 1980s was that it was not just external bodies and individuals who were kept at a distance from the policy process, but the Minister himself who – by choice presumably – played no major public role in the process and, at times, indicated that he was opposed to the introduction of such policy change.

The only official policy document to be published during this phasing in of harm-reduction practices was the *Government Strategy to Prevent Drug Misuse* (1991),[26] which was ostensibly the work of the reconstituted National Co-ordinating Committee on Drug Abuse. However, many of the senior civil servants appointed to it could not be expected to have had a detailed knowledge of the drugs scene, and some of them were replaced during the course of their work on this document. The report itself seems to have been prompted by the necessity to have a national drugs plan, comparable to that being prepared by other European countries, and it is difficult to resist the conclusion that its content and style were primarily dictated by Department of Health officials. In its content, this 1991 report did not attempt to grapple with the policy dilemma posed by HIV/AIDS or to discuss in detail what harm reduction entailed. In a critique written soon after its publication, this author (Butler, 1991) drew the following conclusion:

> Viewed in the context of Irish drug policy and practice over the past twenty five years, this report cannot be seen, however, as marking a radical departure. It is, in its overall tone, an administrator's report rather than a policy maker's report. It is, even more than the 1971 *Report of the Working Party on Drug Abuse*, concerned with closing down rather than opening up a debate, and with making arrangements rather than considering alternative policy positions. Given that for more than twenty years Irish drug policy was concerned with total abstinence and the achievement of a drug-free society, one might expect a full discussion of the policy changes which are contained in this new strategy. No such discussion is provided, however, and the phrase 'harm reduction' occurs just once in the main text.[27]

The re-constituted National Co-ordinating Committee on Drug Abuse fared no better than its predecessors and, following the publication of just one report, appeared to exist only in name.

At one level, it could be argued that the tendency of departmental officials to keep their own counsel and to control policy events, rather than promoting public debate and participative decision-making, was functional from a health promotion perspective. Viewed in this light, the Department of Health had used its well-established political skills to introduce strategies which offered a good chance of reducing HIV transmission, and in so doing had further highlighted the naïveté and lack of such skills on the part of the Health Education Bureau. It would be unusual, however, if a policy process of this type – the very antithesis of the WHO's ideal type of health promotion policy – delivered consistently positive outcomes from a health promotional perspective, and some of the negative consequences of this covert and incremental style of policy making will now be considered.

In order to tease out these negative consequences, it is necessary to restate some of the defining features of harm reduction which were presented earlier in this chapter. The most important point, perhaps, was that harm reduction did not simply entail the introduction of practices which promised to reduce the risk of HIV transmission, but that it also – at least implicitly – reflected a view of drug users which no longer was based solely on notions of pathology and deviance. The new view of drug users as health service consumers was one which ideally saw them as having strengths and competence, and as being uniquely well placed to advise on how risk might be reduced; they were to be seen as active collaborators with healthcare professionals in the task of HIV prevention, rather than as passive recipients of services delivered by professionals, on terms dictated by professionals.

In Dublin, however, because new strategies were surreptitiously introduced into the healthcare system, it was not just the opponents of harm reduction who were confused by this turn of events but also the service providers themselves. No new philosophy was enunciated and no formal training programmes set in place to bring about a change of minds and hearts in practitioners for whom the abstinence model was an article of faith. One way in which this confusion manifested itself was in the situation of newly recruited outreach workers for the Eastern Health Board's AIDS Resource Centre, who wondered if what they were doing in taking needles and syringes out of the centre was legal and in accordance with Health Board policy.[28] The greatest difficulty, however, arose in relation to the new National Drug Treatment Centre Board, which had relocated from its original base in Jervis Street Hospital to premises in Pearse Street, which were called 'Trinity Court'.

What appears to have happened was that harm reduction practices were introduced into (if not imposed upon) an existing service without any attempt at bringing about philosophical or attitudinal changes in long-serving staff. There was, therefore, a great disparity between practice and philosophy, which was problematic for both service consumers and professional service providers. Drug users attending the Trinity Court service tended to complain that despite the availability of methadone maintenance (and later of needle exchange), attitudes of staff were still moralistic and authoritarian; instead of offering an opportunity for constructive partnership, methadone sometimes appeared to become a source of conflict between service users and service providers. One HIV-positive woman, in a research interview during 1989, expressed her views about Trinity Court in the following terms:

> The only reason they are concerned about us now is because they think that if they keep us from using, then we won't spread the virus ... It was hard to get on the maintenance programme and it seems even harder now. I don't know if it's that they're too busy and can't cope. There are no fresh ideas ... When you can stand up for yourself they can't stand it. A lot of addicts going there live for their Phy (methadone) and are terrified.[29]

One striking public example of how staff attitudes had remained unchanged was to be seen in a 1989 paper by Peggy Comberton, Senior Social Worker at Trinity Court, in an issue of the *Irish Social Worker* devoted to AIDS. In this special issue, Peggy Comberton and Joan Cronin (a social worker who was employed at this time in the Ana Liffey Drug Project) took opposing sides in a debate on the merits of needle exchange. In her paper, Joan Cronin outlined the harm-reduction rationale for needle exchange, and referred briefly to the preliminary – and generally positive – evaluative research on British needle exchange schemes. Peggy Comberton was unequivocal in her denunciation of needle exchange, and indeed of harm reduction generally, arguing that those who advocated harm reduction did so from a position of ignorance. 'It would appear', she wrote, 'that there are too few people expert in the field of addiction involved in analysing the situation and AIDS prevention planning.' She then went on to provide the following 'profile' of a heroin addict:

> It would be useful, therefore to look at a profile of a heroin addict: he lives in a cocoon of his own making, of denial, delusion and avoidance. Contact with others is mainly to manipulate them into giving him what he wants. These usually include his parents, wife/husband, boy/girlfriend, GPs and others who do not understand addiction. He, of course, exploits relationships and situations, lies with great ease and blames everyone, his parents, agencies, hospitals, society, etc., for his situation and difficulties. He takes NO responsibility for his own life or what he does ...[30]

It is understandable that a long-serving social worker, with experience in Jervis Street and in Trinity Court, should hold views of this kind; these, after all, were the conceptualisations of drug users which had underpinned this centralised type of service provision since its inception in 1969. Nobody had publicly challenged the validity of such views of drug users or questioned their helpfulness from a practical perspective,[31] but obviously these were not views which were compatible with partnership approaches to working with drug users or which readily lent themselves to the development of specific harm-reduction initiatives such as peer support networks. This latter concept of 'peer support' refers to the training and employment of current drug users in a health promotion and social support role amongst their peers, a concept which had been particularly associated with Dutch drug policy prior to the advent of HIV, and which clearly implies that drug users cannot be described in the categorically negative terms used by Peggy Comberton.

During the second half of the 1980s, therefore, specific harm reduction practices were introduced into the Jervis Street/Trinity Court drug treatment centre in an attempt to stop the transmission of HIV amongst its clients. These changes were proposed by Department of Health officials (and most notably, it would appear, by Dr James Walsh, the National AIDS Co-ordinator) who were specifically concerned with HIV/AIDS, rather than by the moribund National Co-ordinating Committee on Drug Abuse. However, in the absence of an official announcement of a policy revision or a staff retraining scheme to accompany and support the newly introduced harm-reduction practices, it appeared that the agency as a whole had not shifted philosophically or attitudinally in its perception of clients. On the contrary, some Trinity Court staff at least regarded harm reduction as being in violation of the value systems which had previously underpinned their practice, and they expressed genuine and understandable qualms about the morality of these new practices.

What also added to the difficulties of working in Trinity Court during this period was the fact that clients were increasingly familiar with what was happening in the British drug treatment scene at this time and were not slow to compare the Trinity Court ethos with that prevailing in Britain. Sometimes these comparisons were made publicly, as in August 1989 when the *Irish Times* carried a feature on this topic. Dr Michael Farrell, a Dublin-born psychiatrist who specialised in drug treatment in London, was quoted at length on what he saw as the desirable policy changes which now characterised British services:

> 'They (the drug services) are developing a more user-friendly, accessible service … There must be an emphasis on harm reduction, an emphasis on people altering drug using behaviour so that they're not transmitting hepatitis B or HIV. We're talking about a new public health model of drugs services. We're talking about a health conscious drug user. They are like most people, they don't want to die,' says Dr Farrell.[32]

Accompanying this was a reported account of his treatment at Trinity Court by a Dublin drug user named Seán; this young man was living in London at the time he spoke to *The Irish Times* and his comparison of the ethos of the London drug treatment system with that of Trinity Court was presented under the headline 'In Ireland they treat you like a scumbag'.[33] He conceded that methadone maintenance had been available to him when he was last in Dublin, but, like the woman cited earlier in this section, he was highly critical of staff attitudes and of the general regime at Trinity Court. He concluded:

> Seeing is believing and you would want to see Trinity Court on a Saturday morning. Everyone has to be there before 12.30pm to get their methadone. I mean, it's like a cattle market. It's just a methadone feeding station, that's all it is, a methadone feeding station.[34]

Finally, it can also be argued that the covert transition to harm reduction described here delayed the introduction of localised services, through its failure to produce clear and explicit guidelines on such contentious issues as the respective roles of the Eastern Health Board (the statutory health authority for the Dublin area) and the National Drug Treatment Centre, or on the role of GPs in the management of drug users. The difficulties which surrounded the establishment of locally-based services and the creation of a clearer role for GPs in this somewhat confused policy climate will now be looked at in some detail.

Creating community-based services for opiate users

While generally recommending a shift away from centralised drug treatment systems, the 1991 *Government Strategy to Prevent Drug Misuse* neither acknowledged nor presented a detailed approach to the difficulties entailed in such a shift. Instead, somewhat equivocally, this report proposed a greater role for the Eastern Health Board in the development of community drug services in Dublin (including more involvement of general practitioners), while at the same time recommending 'a strengthening of the role of the Drug Treatment Centre, Trinity Court, and an expansion of the Board membership'.[35]

This change to the Board membership in Trinity Court did not immediately improve matters, however, and for the five years (1991-1996) following the publication of the strategy document the relationship between Trinity Court and the Eastern Health Board continued to be uneasy and confused. The policy differences between these two institutions were symbolised to some extent in the differing backgrounds of two of their key players. Dr John O'Connor, the Clinical Director of Trinity Court, was a consultant psychiatrist specialising in addictions, accustomed to a good deal of professional autonomy and apparently sceptical of the value of harm reduction.[36] On the other hand, Dr Joe Barry, who acted as AIDS/Drugs Co-ordinator for the Eastern Health Board during this period, was a specialist in public health medicine, primarily interested in HIV prevention and pragmatically well-disposed towards harm reduction.[37]

Attempts by the Eastern Health Board to involve general practitioners in the medical management of drug users also proved to be slow and complicated. It could, of course, be argued that regardless of the style of policy making, this was always going to be a difficult task; the general but implicit view for twenty years prior to the coming of HIV was that GPs should simply refer problem drug users to the national treatment centre, on the basis that methadone prescribing by GPs would be uncontrolled and would inevitably result in leakage of this drug on to the black market. The 1991 *Government Strategy to Prevent Drug Misuse* contained two specific recommendations as to how GPs could be effectively drawn into the medical management of problem drug users. One of these borrowed from British service developments in this area in its proposal for 'the development of Community Drug Teams under the auspices of the Health Boards to operate with the involvement of General Practitioners and other health professionals in targeted areas'.[38]

While the Eastern Health Board appeared to have become somewhat disenchanted with the national Drug Treatment Centre and to have placed more reliance on its own efforts to develop community services, its track record of collaboration with community-based professionals and local activists (as discussed in detail in Chapter Six) was poor, and it could not be presumed that it would readily develop the capacity to change and improve in this regard. It would therefore have been helpful if the 1991 strategy document had been more detailed and elaborate in its depiction of the philosophy and methods of the Community Drug Team (CDT) rather than confining itself to a brief and uncritical account of what the creation of CDTs entailed. It was not altogether surprising, therefore, that the first attempt by the Eastern Health Board to set up a CDT should have ended as badly as it did. This first venture was based in Ballymun, and consisted of a formal partnership between the Eastern Health Board and a voluntary body, the Ballymun Youth Action Project. The Ballymun CDT was set up in 1992, only to be dissolved in 1995 in a flurry of mutual recriminations which was reminiscent of earlier relationships between the health board and locally based drugs groupings. Conflict between the partner agencies may have been partly attributable to ideological differences in relation to harm-reduction, about which the Youth Action Project was less enthusiastic then the Eastern Health Board, but the report of an independent evaluator suggested that one of the fundamental difficulties with this project was confusion as to what a CDT was or how the two participating agencies were to collaborate. Something of the intensity of the bad feeling and confusion involved may be gleaned from the following comments of the project's evaluator:

> It is essential that both partners are clear about why they are in partnership, what they wish to achieve and how they will do so. This evaluation has shown that such clarity did not exist, that the vision, aims etc., did not go much beyond general statements of aspiration, that the partners did not openly share their agendas for being in partnership, that they guessed at each other's motivation for being in partnership and never checked out their assumptions, that there were so many differing expectations of the CDT which were never articulated and dealt with and which ultimately resulted in inactivity, frustration and anger.[39]

Following the breakdown of the Ballymun pilot project, the Eastern Health Board appeared to lose its enthusiasm for the CDT concept. The new determination of the EHB to develop community-based drug services, which appeared to be a radical reversal of its policy during the period of the 'opiate epidemic', was greatly complicated in the 1990s both by its own inexperience in negotiating with local community groups and by the ambivalence of these local groups towards problem drug users. Typically, what happened between 1991 and 1996 was that local community groups which experienced drug use as seriously disruptive of their neighbourhoods started to campaign for 'something to be done'; such campaigning involved lobbying of constituency TDs and local authority representatives as well as direct lobbying of the EHB. However, when the EHB responded to such lobbying by attempting to set up local services, the communities involved often expressed great antagonism to the siting of treatment facilities in their areas. The phrase 'not in my back-yard' (commonly abbreviated as NIMBY) was frequently used with reference to such communal ambivalence on this subject. One striking example of this NIMBY phenomenon occurred during 1995 when, in response to local agitation for the creation of a drug treatment service in Blanchardstown in west Dublin, the EHB attempted to open a methadone clinic in the gate lodge of James Connolly Memorial Hospital in Blanchardstown. This plan was greeted with great hostility by local residents who mounted a picket on the premises, and it was only after months of conflict that a resolution was achieved – involving a climb-down by the health board on its proposal for a methadone clinic in this premises.

When it came to creating community-based drug treatment services, therefore, health board officials and professionals tended to see themselves as trapped in a no-win situation, as did elected public representatives. Local community groups complained about the negative impact which untreated drug use was having on their neighbourhoods, yet rejected the establishment of what the authorities saw as appropriate local services. It was abundantly clear that ideas about community participation and community empowerment, such as those contained in the Ottawa Charter, were rather naïve and superficial when applied to partnership or collaborative activities between statutory health authorities and local neighbourhood groupings on the drugs issue. The involvement of local residents and community activists in the provision of treatment services was not an entirely benign affair devoted to the welfare of drug users, but tended to be characterised by huge ambivalence, with aggression towards or rejection of drug users as a regular feature of such activity. As concluded in Chapter Six, this situation could be interpreted as justifying and vindicating the scepticism of the Eastern Health Board about community participation in drug services and as confirming the Board's belief in the superiority of professionalism. Alternatively, in the light of this extended discussion of covert and incremental policy shifts, it could be seen that local antagonism towards drug users merely reflected the ambivalence of the Eastern Health Board's own position on this issue, as well as the difficulties which might be expected when quite radical changes were introduced into the treatment system without open discussion and elaborate re-training schemes.

One of the specific recommendation of the *Government Strategy to Prevent Drug Misuse* (1991) was for 'the development of a greater role for General Practitioners in the treatment of drug misuse at community level with the central support of the Drug Treatment Centre'.[40] Again, the rather cursory treatment of this topic in the strategy document, and the failure to tease out the policy issues associated with such an initiative, meant that its implementation was unlikely to be a speedy and trouble-free business. The phrase 'a greater role for General Practitioners' was interpreted by many close to these issues as a code to describe the expansion of methadone maintenance prescribing by GPs, and there were two main difficulties which could be anticipated in this scheme. The first was that many GPs appeared to share the common negative perceptions of drug users as devious, manipulative and aggressive, on which basis they were unwilling to become involved in their treatment. The second difficulty was the fear that GPs might prescribe excessive amounts of methadone for individual patients, which would lead to leakage on to the black market, and also that the black market for methadone would be supplied by drug users who would simply attend several doctors at one time and accumulate a supply for illicit sale. In Britain, as will be recalled from Chapters Five and Six, the debate as to whether GP prescribing of maintenance drugs was a good or a bad thing had been concerned with precisely these issues, and with the merits of allowing GPs a high degree of clinical freedom in this matter as opposed to confining maintenance prescribing to specialists based in centralised services. While it could not be said that British policy makers had achieved any resolution of this dilemma, at least it could be said of the British situation that the issues had been clearly identified, discussed and researched over a considerable period. In Ireland, by contrast, these issues had never been publicly debated and it had always been assumed that GP prescribing of drugs such as methadone was more likely to do harm than good.

However, through the work of a small number of GPs who were committed to treating drug users, the Irish College of General Practitioners (ICGP) prepared and circulated a policy document on this topic in 1990.[41] This policy statement argued that GPs had a legitimate role in this field, while at the same time recommending that they should not work in isolation with such patients but should instead work collaboratively with other appropriate health and social services. While it would be naïve to interpret this statement as reflecting a broad consensus within the ICGP, it did help considerably to push ahead incrementally with the process of institutionalising methadone prescribing in general medical practice, and in 1992 the Minister for Health established an Expert Group to draw up a formal protocol which would govern methadone prescribing in community services. The Expert Group was chaired by Dr James Walsh who was the National AIDS Co-ordinator at the Department of Health, and the group was convened under the aegis of the National AIDS Strategy Committee rather then as part of the National Co-ordinating Committee on Drug Abuse.[42] Both in terms of its membership and its style of working – which will now be looked at in some detail – the appointment of this Expert Group suggested that harm reduction was now being taken seriously and that the policy process was shifting more towards an organisational networks model.

The Expert Group carried out its task of considering 'methadone prescribing, registration of drug users and licensing of general practitioners to treat drug users'[43] quietly and discreetly, consulting only with the Irish College of General Practitioners, the Pharmaceutical Society of Ireland and the Pharmaceutical Union. The group concluded its work in March 1993, recommending that methadone be used for maintenance purposes and in many ways reiterating the views of the ICGP as to what constituted good practice in this field. It decided not to recommend that the right to prescribe methadone be legally restricted to specially licensed GPs, largely, it said, because it anticipated opposition to such a scheme from doctors' representative organisations, but compromised on this issue of GP autonomy by recommending that patients should be assessed by either Trinity Court or the health board specialist addiction service before starting on a maintenance programme with a GP. The Expert Group displayed both political and linguistic skills in dealing with the question of registering maintained addicts. It noted that there was resistance to the use of the term 'register', but then went on to recommend what was effectively a registration system, namely the issuing of an identifying 'treatment card' for all such patients and the creation of a central treatment list.[44]

The same tensions between Trinity Court and the Eastern Health Board which have already been noted also manifested themselves in the workings of this Expert Group, with Dr John O'Connor of the former institution expressing reservations about developing a greater role for GPs in methadone maintenance. Dr O'Connor's reservations on this subject are clearly evident in a short paper, *Good Clinical Practice in Relation to Methadone Prescribing*, which he prepared for the Expert Group and which is included as an appendix to the group's report; his final caveat was expressed in terms of his belief that 'Methadone should always be regarded as an adjunct to treatment and not treatment per se'.[45]

Considered in terms of formal models of policy analysis, the work of the Expert Group is probably best seen, as stated above, as an example of the organisational networks model, with those civil servants in the Department of Health who were now committed to harm reduction playing a key role as co-ordinators of this network. Having made this commitment to harm reduction, it has to be said that the civil servants displayed considerable skill and patience in managing its introduction into a policy environment which was somewhat hostile to such beliefs and practices. Following the completion of the Expert Group's report, it lay unpublicised and unpublished for three years, presumably because the civil servants most involved judged that the time was not right to launch any bold initiative on this front. It is interesting to note, for example, that in February 1993 – as the Expert Group was completing its report and at a time when Eastern Health Board local clinics and harm-reduction services were reasonably well established – Councillor Joe Connolly, a member of the EHB, received considerable publicity for his suggestion at a board meeting that drug addicts should be summarily rounded up by the army and detained. *The Evening Herald*, which gave this story banner headlines on its front page, reported it thus:

> An unrepentant Dublin councillor today defended his call that soldiers be used to round up addicts. 'This is war,' said Eastern Health Board member Joe Connolly. Insisting that emergency measures were needed to deal with drugs, Councillor Connolly urged army patrols escort addicts off the streets for hospital treatment … 'The army don't need powers of arrest to do this. Drug addicts are sick people, "Jekyll and Hyde" characters who become evil at night when they get drugs. It would be doing them a favour. We have to keep them off the streets.'[46]

These views of Councillor Connolly had no appreciable impact on EHB policy and service structures, but the mere fact that he expressed them suggests that board members had no detailed appreciation of harm reduction at this time in 1993.

It could be argued perhaps that during this protracted policy process more could have been done to build public support for having GPs involved in methadone maintenance; certainly, when the new protocol was being set up on a pilot basis in early 1996, little progress appeared to have been made on this front. The RTÉ news programme *Prime Time* did a lengthy and balanced feature on methadone maintenance on 15 February, 1996, which revealed that there was still widespread opposition to this approach to drug treatment. Furthermore, the *Sunday Business Post* of 18 February, 1996, had a comment or editorial piece which was scathing in its criticism of *Prime Time* and what it saw as the unproven assumptions which underpinned the programme's case for methadone maintenance. In part, this editorial piece read as follows:

> We believe that the central assumptions and theses of this programme are entirely unproven, and it was quite wrong to broadcast it in the manner in which it was transmitted … People suffering from addiction to substances such as heroin and vodka do have a fundamental right. That right is best exercised by the provision of help which, in large measure, comes in forms other than the substance which is being abused. That is to say, they should be helped to recover their physical strength and their self-esteem to regain their place in society. This will not be achieved by the creation of ghettoes of state-financed drug addiction.[47]

This hostility of the *Sunday Business Post* towards methadone maintenance can be regarded as further evidence of the negative side of covert policy-making. What the editorial was objecting to was what it saw as a policy *fait accompli,* and, ironically, it is likely that had there been a detailed and lengthy policy debate on methadone, the *Sunday Business Post* (with its conservative economic views) would have been persuaded that this particular form of treatment was cost effective.

As with the general introduction of harm reduction into Ireland, the avoidance of public debate and heated controversy on the subject of GP treatment of opiate users facilitated service developments which might otherwise have never taken place in a conservative political culture. The negative aspects of this covert style of policy making by small networks are also clear, however. The introduction of harm-reduction strategies was by normal standards a protracted affair, which frustrated those committed to harm reduction and lengthened the period of time during which injecting drug users were at greater risk of HIV infection. The failure to spell out in detail the philosophical underpinnings of harm reduction meant that negative stereotypical views of drug users persisted, despite the utilisation of new strategies, and also that health authorities and health care professionals were slow to come to terms with partnership or collaborative models of working with local community or other interest groups.

1996 – a year of transition

If 1996 was an eventful year for alcohol policy, it was also an interesting and significant year for Irish drug policy. A number of specific developments in drug policy took place during 1996 which generally suggested that there was now a greater willingness to make the policy process more visible than it had been prior to this.

In October 1995 the Minister for Health had announced that the Eastern Health Board was to set up a new management sub-structure specifically designed to deal with the complexities of drug treatment and rehabilitation. This was done immediately and the EHB's new drug management team went on to conduct a review of its work in this field during 1995 and to prepare a development plan for 1996. Two external reviewers, the British-based psychiatrist Dr Michael Farrell, and a Dutch psychologist, Ernst Buning, were commissioned to do an assessment of the EHB's drug services, and their report – which reaffirmed the therapeutic value of methadone maintenance and was generally affirmatory and encouraging of EHB community service developments – was included in the plan which was prepared for a Special Board Meeting on 2 April, 1996.[48] The Eastern Health Board's plan for 1996 contained ten specific proposals for expanding its drug treatment services, the most ambitious of which was for an increase in the number of methadone maintenance places available from 1,400 to 2,500; this increase was to take place through a range of service and facility options, including new clinics, further involvement of GPs and the use of a mobile clinic. The EHB appeared to be buoyed up by the positive tone of the external reviewers' report and to be facing into the future with a degree of clarity and self-confidence that it had not previously displayed.

The 1996 development plan also reported that two new consultant psychiatrist posts in drug services had been established and that, with the inclusion of Dr O'Connor from Trinity Court, this had facilitated the division of the EHB's region into three catchment areas for the service delivery purposes. This, on the face of it, was a most important innovation which appeared to signal the end of Trinity Court's role as an independent centralised service and a victory of sorts for the Eastern Health Board in its struggle to change the philosophy of drug treatment services which had existed since the establishment of the drugs unit at Jervis Street Hospital in 1969. However, the National Drug Treatment Centre Board had not been abolished, and the EHB report contained no detailed information or underlying rationale bearing on this new arrangement. Furthermore, the two external reviewers did not attempt any analysis of the organisational confusion which still characterised relationships between the Eastern Health Board and Trinity Court. The EHB's drug service plan appeared to be generally well received, or at least it could be said that it did not evoke any strongly negative public reactions.

Another highly significant policy development took place in early October 1996 with the publication of the *First Report of the Ministerial Task Force on Measures to Reduce the Demand for Drugs*. This Task Force had a membership of seven Ministers of State under the chair of Pat Rabbitte, Minister of State to the Government, with representation from Education, Health, Justice, Social Welfare and the Environment; it had been established in July 1996 'to review the present arrangements for a co-ordinated approach to drugs demand reduction and, in the light of the review, to identify for Governmental Action any changes or additional measures needed to provide a more effective response to the problem'.[49] The report of this Ministerial Task Force, which became known colloquially as the 'Rabbitte Report', was, in terms of its presentation and design, somewhat confusing and repetitive; when compared with the *National Alcohol Policy* (see Chapter Four) which was published at approximately the same time, the Rabbitte Report clearly lacked the polish of a policy document which had been compiled slowly, with careful drafting, re-drafting and design work all aimed at enhancing the visual appeal of the final product. Reading through the Rabbitte Report, it becomes clear that all members of the Task Force had fought to stake a claim for their respective departmental sectors and that the resulting document was somewhat fragmented. Despite its confusion, the Rabbitte Report had an immediacy and a directness which was unusual in drug policy documents, and its authors appeared to be genuinely committed to doing something – and doing something quickly – to address Dublin's opiate problem.

Perhaps the most significant conclusion reached by the Ministers of State was that macro-environmental factors were causally significant in Dublin's opiate problem, and that preventive or demand-reduction work should reflect and incorporate this fact. The Rabbitte Report noted that the submissions which it received had consistently 'identified the same underlying causes of problem drug use as had already been identified by the Group, i.e. social disadvantage/exclusion, characterised in high levels of unemployment, poor housing conditions, low educational attainment, lack of recreational facilities, etc'.[50] The primary strategy recommended by the Task Force to deal with this newly acknowledged causal link between social deprivation and serious drug problems was the funding and establishment of eleven *Local Drugs Task Forces* (ten of which were to be in Dublin and one in Cork City). These Local Drugs Task Forces would consist of partnerships between statutory authorities and local community groups, with the intention of using them as a vehicle for targeting resources at areas where there was a high prevalence of problem drug use. The areas in question were designated in the Rabbitte Report and an initial commitment of £10 million was made towards the establishment of Local Drugs Task Forces in these areas. The Report also endorsed the use of methadone on a maintenance basis, and reiterated what had already been said by the Eastern Health Board about the necessity to reduce waiting lists for methadone.

This proposal to establish Local Drugs Task Forces which would selectively target resources at those areas with an identified high prevalence of drug problems was very similar to the proposal of the Special Governmental Task Force (1983) to designate some parts of Dublin as *Community Priority Areas*. However, as discussed in Chapter Six, this earlier proposal had not only been rejected by the Government of the day but had been kept secret, when the report of this 1983 Task Force was effectively suppressed. Some attempt should be made here, therefore, to explain why, thirteen years on, the Government was more amenable to environmental strategies for the prevention or amelioration of drug problems than it had been in 1983, when it had stuck solidly to individualistic explanations and strategies.

Perhaps one explanation for this new willingness to consider environmental approaches, which could broadly be described as community development programmes, was the obvious failure of all previous attempts to reduce the demand for drugs in socially deprived urban communities. Politicians who represented such communities were constantly aware of public criticism of their failure to deal effectively with drug issues, and politicians *en masse* were confronted with the public shock and outrage that followed the murder of the journalist Veronica Guerin in June 1996, apparently by criminals whose main source of income was drug trafficking. While one political response to this murder was to toughen supply-reduction policy, it seems plausible at least to conclude that this shocking event also gave an impetus to demand-reduction policy.

A second explanation for this willingness to set in place Local Drug Task Forces, which would include both *vertical* partnership between statutory authorities and local voluntary and community interests, and *horizontal* or intersectoral partnership between different sectors of the state, can surely be found in the vastly altered approach to social and economic planning which had prevailed from the late 1980s onwards. This approach was broadly characterised as one of social partnership, in which the state co-ordinated a network of the most prominent stakeholders in Irish social and economic life, rather than in terms of the state acting autonomously. The dramatic upsurge in the Irish economy (the so-called 'Celtic tiger') and the relatively peaceful state of the country's industrial relations tended to be largely attributed to the success of the social partnership concept, so that it seemed quite natural that this concept should be extended in this way to community drug policy issues. While there was considerable evidence of conflict between the Eastern Health Board and local community groups, the Task Force pronounced itself 'impressed with the positive impact of the Inter-Agency Drug Project in Dublin's North Inner City'[51] and in many ways used this project as a model upon which to base its proposals for Local Drugs Task Forces. It is also noteworthy that the Rabbitte Report in opting for a partnership approach to resolving drug problems did not draw upon any health promotional literature but instead described this social problem as a 'cross-cutting' issue – a reference to a central tenet of the Strategic Management Initiative (SMI) which pointed out that important public policy objectives were frequently attainable only through inter-sectoral collaboration. In further pursuance of this interest in managing cross-cutting issues, the Ministerial Task Force recommended the establishment of a *National Drugs Strategy Team,* which would consist of representatives of relevant public sector interests as well as community and voluntary representatives. This Strategy Team, which was to report to a new Cabinet Drug Committee, was intended in line with the general philosophy of SMI to institutionalise organisational networking; what it proposed to do was to take senior civil servants out of their parent departments for up to half their working week, thus encouraging them to tackle drug problems as members of an intersectoral team rather than seeing these problems from their traditional 'departmentalist' perspective.

It seems reasonable to conclude, therefore, that while the Rabbitte Report may be seen as health promotional in tenor, it was not explicitly or self-consciously so. It was ironic, however, that a committee comprised of Ministers of State representing a wide cross-section of governmental activities, and chaired by a Minister of State from the Department of the Taoiseach, should ultimately produce a policy report which, in its essence, was closer to health promotion theory than any report previously produced under the aegis of the Department of Health. Referring back to Harrison and Tether's three models of policy co-ordination, which were discussed in Chapter One and which have served as a framework for analysing health policy developments throughout this study, it would seem clear that the third model – *the organisational networks model* – is very similar to the public policy model which now underpins the entire social partnership system. The creation of community development approaches to drug problems in deprived urban areas arose, therefore, from the application of such an organisational network concept by a broadly-based Ministerial group rather than from the application of health promotional concepts to this issue by the Minister or Department of Health.

The final – and some might say the most important – explanation for the content of the Rabbitte Report has already been alluded to: the healthy state of the public purse in 1996, as opposed to the recessionary state of 1983, meant that politicians now had the money to invest in large-scale community development projects. Furthermore, with an impending general election, the politicians who drew up this report were anxious to have their recommendations implemented as speedily as possible so that in the forthcoming election campaign they could claim credit for these new programmes; this obviously meant that the establishment of the Local Drugs Task Forces was pushed forward at a pace dictated by political concerns rather than at the more leisurely pace of the civil service.

Conclusion

The main objective of this chapter was to trace the evolution and adaptation of Irish drug policy between 1986 and 1996, the era of HIV and AIDS. The necessity for change arose initially from the recognition that injecting drug users were infecting one another through the practice of needle sharing and that, through sexual behaviour, such drug use constituted a bridge for the further transmission of HIV into the general population. It was argued that the introduction of pragmatic public health strategies – such as the use of prescribed oral methadone as a heroin substitute, or the provision of sterile injecting equipment through needle exchange schemes – was especially difficult in a policy arena where public debate on drug issues had not been generally encouraged and where it had been previously assumed that all sectors of government were committed to a 'drug-free' society. Aside from this understandable preoccupation with public health issues, the period studied in this chapter may also be seen as one in which, however reluctantly, Irish society was moving towards an acceptance of the fact that illicit drug use was here to stay and that its broader impact, particularly through drug-related crime, demanded some policy adjustments in this country.

Harm reduction strategies which would have previously been regarded as morally dubious were introduced into the Irish healthcare system. This discreet style of policy change – largely based on small organisational networks rather than on the work of the National Co-ordinating Committee on Drug Abuse which had been formally charged with the task of policy making in this sphere – could in many ways be seen as functional since it avoided public controversy and made it difficult for those opposed to harm reduction to have a clear target for their attacks. On the other hand, this style of policy making was dysfunctional in that it did not facilitate attitudinal or philosophical change in long-standing services and personnel; neither did it identify and resolve the confusion which arose between new locally-based services and the existing centralised services.

Throughout this period, 1986-1996, the Department of Health continued to dominate, if not indeed monopolise, the policy process, and it was only in the last year of that decade (1996) that a broad environmental and multi-sectoral strategy for the prevention of drug problems was adopted by a committee in which, ironically, the health sector was not dominant. Many factors contributed to the new approach recommended by the so-called Rabbitte Committee, not least of these being the buoyant state of the national economy. It was also significant, however, that the explicit interest in public policy and management engendered by SMI led to a new recognition of drug problems as 'cross-cutting' issues which demanded appropriate intersectoral solutions.

NOTES
1. *Health: The Wider Dimensions.* (Dublin: Department of Health, 1986), p.26.
2. Male homosexual behaviour had remained a criminal offence in the Republic of Ireland as a result of inherited British legislation, namely the Offences Against the Person Act, 1861. A campaign to have this law reformed was started in 1979 and was headed by a gay activist, David Norris; having failed in the Irish courts, Mr Norris appealed to the European Court of Human Rights which in 1988 ruled that this Irish law was in breach of the European Convention on Human Rights and Fundamental Freedoms. The law in Ireland was not amended, however, until the Criminal Law (Sex Offences) Act, 1993 eventually decriminalised male homosexual behaviour for those over the age of 17.
3. Needle and syringe exchange schemes simply consisted of the provision of new injecting equipment for intravenous drug users so as to eliminate or reduce the practice of sharing such equipment amongst a number of users. Some such schemes operated strictly on the basis of one-for-one exchange, where used 'works' were replaced by old, while other schemes took a more flexible approach.
4. G. Edwards, 'What Drives British Drug Policy?', *British Journal of Addiction,* 84 (1989), p.223.
5. For a systematic review of outreach work see T. Rhodes, *Outreach work with drug users: principles and practice.* (Strasbourg: Council of Europe, 1996).

6.   E. Engelsman, 'Dutch Policy on the Management of Drug-Related Problems', *British Journal of Addiction,* 84 (1989), pp 211-218.

7.   Health Education Bureau, *Teacher Training Programme in Health Education.* (Dublin: Health Education Bureau, no date).

8.   D. Manly, L. Browne, G. Cox, and P. Lowry, *The Facilitators.* (Dublin: Brandsma Books, 1986); J. McCarroll, *Is the School Around the Corner Just the Same?.* (Dublin: Brandsma Books, 1987).

9.   K. McNamara, *Curriculum and Values in Education.* (Dublin: Veritas, 1987): J. Newman, *Puppets of Utopia: can Irish democracy be taken for granted?* (Dublin: Four Courts Press, 1987).

10.   *The Ballintrillick Review* (Autumn 1987), p.12.

11.   *First Annual Report of the National Co-ordinating Committee on Drug Abuse.* (Dublin: Stationery Office, 1986).

12.   Ibid., p. 21.

13.   One senior civil servant subsequently confirmed the validity of this interpretation in an informal discussion with this writer in 1993. He admitted that he found the task of working with the committee frustrating, and he preferred to make policy decisions himself.

14.   Advisory Council on the Misuse of Drugs, *AIDS and Drug Misuse (Part 1).* (London: HMSO, 1988).

15.   *Seanad Éireann Debates* (Vol.118), Column 1846.

16.   Ibid., Column 1842.

17.   Ibid., Column 2082.

18.   Ibid., Column 1831.

19.   *Irish Times,* 18 November, 1988.

20.   D. Nutbeam, V. Blakey and R. Pates, 'The Prevention of HIV Infection from Injecting Drug Use – A Review of Health Promotion Approaches', *Social Science and Medicine,* 33 (1991), p.978.

21.   J. Comberton, *The Self-Fulfilling Prophesty* [sic] *of Physeptone Maintenance(1).* (Dublin: Coolemine Programme Information Sheet, no date). This pamphlet was circulated by Coolemine in the early 1980s. 'Physeptone' was the proprietary name of the methadone most commonly used in Dublin at this time.

22.   J. Comberton, *Ireland's Young People Have a Right to a Drug-Free Life.* (Dublin: Coolemine Unpublished Paper, 1990), p.9.

23.   Ibid., p. 12.

24.   Ibid., p. 13.

25.   *Irish Medical Times,* 13 October, 1989.

26.   *Government Strategy to Prevent Drug Misuse.* (Dublin: Department of Health, 1991).

27.   S. Butler, 'Drug Problems and Drug Policies in Ireland: A Quarter of a Century Reviewed', *Administration,* 39 (1991), p.229.

28.   Some former students of Diploma in Addiction Studies in Trinity College Dublin expressed misgivings of this kind to this writer.

29.   S. Butler and M. Woods, 'Drugs, HIV and Ireland: Responses to Women in Dublin' in N. Dorn, S. Henderson and N. South (eds), *AIDS: Women, Drugs and Social Care.* (London: Falmer Press, 1992), pp 63-64.

30. P. Comberton, 'Drug Addiction and AIDS', *The Irish Social Worker*, 8 (1), (1989), pp 9-10.

31. No scientific evidence in support of this negative perception of the personalities of drug users has ever been adduced. O'Mahony and Smith (1984), for example, compared the personality characteristics of heroin addicts in Mountjoy Prison with those of non heroin-using prisoners and a normal control group of civil servants from the Department of Justice. No difference was found in the propensity for self-deception between any of these groups.
P. O'Mahony and E. Smith, 'Some Personality Characteristics of Imprisoned Heroin Addicts', *Drug and Alcohol Dependence 13* (1984), pp 255-265.

32. *Irish Times*, 8 August, 1989.

33. Ibid.

34. Ibid.

35. *Government Strategy to Prevent Drug Misuse.* (Dublin: Department of Health, 1991), p.2.

36. See, for instance, J. O'Connor, 'Is methadone maintenance the answer in drug misuse?', *Irish Medical Times,* 4 March, 1994.

37. See, for instance, Dr Barry's editorial in *AIDS /Drugs News.* (First edition of an Eastern Health Board newsletter, May 1993).

38. *Government Strategy to Prevent Drug Misuse,* cit.sup., p.2.

39. C. Forrestal, *Evaluation Report on Ballymun Community Drug Team.* (Dublin: Community Action Network, 1996), p.36.

40. *Government Strategy to Prevent Drug Misuse,* cit.sup., p.2.

41. Irish College of General Practitioners, *Policy Statement on Illicit Drug Use and Problems of Addiction,* 1990.

42. *Report of the Expert Group on the Establishment of a Protocol for the Prescribing of Methadone.* (Dublin: Department of Health, 1993).
The chair of this committee was Dr James Walsh, National AIDS Co-ordinator, Department of Health, and its other members were : Dr Joe Barry, Drugs/AIDS Co-ordinator, Eastern Health Board; Mr Tony Geoghegan, Project Leader, Merchants Quay Project; Dr Fergus O'Kelly, Irish College of General Practitioners; Dr John O'Connor, Clinical Director, National Drug Treatment Centre, Trinity Court; Dr Brion Sweeney, Consultant Psychiatrist, Eastern Health Board; Mr Dermot Ryan, Department of Health, secretary to the committee.

43. *Report of the Expert Group on the Establishment of a Protocol for the Prescribing of Methadone,* cit. sup., p. 2. The terms of reference of the committee were not spelt out more formally than this.

44. Ibid., pp 8-11.

45. Ibid., p. 18.

46. *Evening Herald,* 12 February, 1993.

47. *Sunday Business Post,* 18 February, 1996.

48. *Drug Service – Review of 1995 and Development Plans for 1996.* (Document prepared for special board meeting of Eastern Health Board, 2 April, 1996).

49. *First Report of the Ministerial Task Force on Measures to Reduce the Demand for Drugs.* (Dublin: Department of the Taoiseach, 1996), p.4.

50. Ibid., p.33.

51. Ibid., p.45.

8

Alcohol, Drugs and Health Promotion in Modern Ireland: A Conclusion

Introduction

Health promotion is a policy perspective which has been developed by the World Health Organisation (WHO), implicitly at first but since the 1970s in an increasingly explicit and public manner. In many ways, this perspective reflects the disillusionment with conventional biomedical practices and institutions which has grown since the middle of the twentieth century: its proponents argue that society has developed a misplaced and exaggerated trust in medicine and in 'high-tech' health care systems dominated by the medical profession.[1] Health promotion has emerged, therefore, as an alternative set of beliefs and practices which attempts to redress the balance by demoting curative medicine from its dominant position and replacing it – or at least complementing it – with a renewed emphasis on disease prevention and on supporting and maintaining good health. For many authors, health promotion is synonymous with 'the new public health',[2] a reference back to the 'old' public health – the major nineteenth-century reforms which radically improved public health in urban areas through environmental measures, such as clean water supplies, sanitation, food hygiene and better housing standards. Thus, it is argued, morbidity and mortality rates in the latter half of the nineteenth century were reduced through diverse measures aimed at environmental change, rather than as a result of specific technical developments in medicine or surgery. It would be an exaggeration of conventional health promotion belief or rhetoric to suggest that it has totally turned its back on curative medicine; rather would it be more accurate to say that health promotion attempts to bring the emphasis back to primary health care – away from what might be seen as an over-reliance on hospital medicine with its trappings of medical specialism and sophisticated technology.

Health promotion policy, as it has evolved from the middle of the twentieth century and particularly as it has been espoused by the WHO, has obvious parallels with its nineteenth-century counterpart: foremost among these is its belief that improvements in human health are more likely to result from broad environmental measures than from better resourced or more technically effective health sector interventions. For health promotionists, however, the concept of environment is considerably broader than that espoused by their nineteenth-century forebears. For the Victorian reformers 'environment' referred simply to the physical habitat, especially those urban neighbourhoods which were seen as inimical to human health. For present-day health promotionists the notion of 'environment' has been extended to incorporate a complex host of social, cultural, political and economic issues. The concept of 'community' has a central place in this new public health, as do the related concepts of 'participation' and 'empowerment'. In summary, it is argued that ordinary people (ordinary in the sense that they are lay people, not healthcare professionals) have an important role to play in creating and sustaining 'health promoting environments' in their own neighbourhoods or communities. It is commonly implied, and sometimes stated explicitly, that there is a moral imperative on the part of these ordinary people to participate in creating and working on a health agenda for their communities; and it is also emphasised that health authorities should 'empower' such participation where communities are prevented by poverty, political disenfranchisement or other factors from such participation in health promotion. The health promotion ideal, therefore, is one of partnership or collaboration between health professionals and the laity, as opposed to the previous tradition which consigned non-professionals to a relatively passive and subordinate role in healthcare matters.

While health promotion has a much greater emphasis on collective or communal activity than is the norm in conventional biomedicine, it also has its own distinctive viewpoint on the importance of individual behaviour or 'lifestyle' for morbidity and mortality. Individuals, it is argued, contribute significantly to shaping their own health status through the choices which they make in terms of food consumption, exercise, sleeping patterns and sexual behaviour, as well of course as their choices in relation to alcohol and drug use. This emphasis on individual behaviour and its importance for health is balanced, however, by an equal emphasis on the central role of structural or environmental factors in shaping individual choices, so that health promotionists seek to avoid the worst excesses of naïve individualism, an individualism which could easily degenerate into a form of 'victim blaming'. It is recognised that not all social contexts or environments are equally conducive to health, and so policy is directed at changing the environment with a view to 'making the healthier choice the easier choice'.[3]

From a policy-making perspective, health promotion differs radically from traditional health policy in its insistence that real improvements in the health status of a society cannot be solely reliant on the health sector of government. Instead, it is argued that all public policy has health implications and that public health can only be effectively promoted through the conscious collaboration of all governmental sectors; this intersectoral collaboration is aimed at bringing about what health promotionists describe as 'healthy public policy'. While the health promotion agenda may generally be seen as an ambitious one, this specific aspect of it, which envisages the health sector as securing the co-operation of all other governmental sectors, seems particularly ambitious and difficult to realise.

The above account of health promotion, much of which was summarised under the rubric of the *Ottawa Charter* in Chapter One, sets the scene for a final analysis of what has been presented and discussed in the preceding seven chapters. The policy document *Health: The Wider Dimensions,* which was published by the Department of Health in 1986, was the first explicit and detailed exposition of health promotion by Irish statutory authorities. As noted in Chapter One, this document concluded its account of health promotion and its applicability to Ireland with the suggestion that: 'The cynical and fatalistic will probably dismiss such an approach as a grand design incapable of being achieved'. The findings of the present study indicate that during the period studied Irish health policy on alcohol and illicit drugs made some, but not a great deal of, progress in the realisation of health promotional aspirations. Whether these findings warrant the description 'cynical and fatalistic' is a moot point, but they certainly confirm the naïvete of those who aspire to a 'grand design' without spelling out in detail how such a design can be achieved. It would seem fair to conclude that proponents of health promotion have generally failed to pay as much attention to policy strategies as they have to the statement and reiteration of their aspirations; by and large, they have succeeded in making clear *what* it is they wish to achieve, while largely ignoring the question of *how* these radical aspirations are to be attained.

Alcohol, illicit drugs and healthy public policy

If health promotion were to move beyond rhetoric and become a reality, it would have to confront and shape a socio-cultural environment infinitely more complex than the physical environment which was successfully tackled by the public health reformers of the nineteenth century. One of the main advantages of using two similar, though subtly different, case studies in this book is that it allows for a more detailed analysis of the difficulties faced by the health sector in challenging the *status quo,* in cultural, economic and political matters, than would be possible if just one of these topics had been studied. It may be argued from an objective biomedical perspective that the similarities between the consumption of alcohol and the consumption of illicit drugs greatly outweigh the dissimilarities: each may be considered in terms of toxicity and associated long-term or short-term health risk; each may be considered in terms of potential for addiction or dependency; and each may be considered in terms of impact on the behaviour or personality of individual users and what might be considered the knock-on effects on society. However, the findings of this study demonstrate clearly that Irish health policy has not been moving towards the creation of a unitary, rational, or research-based, substance abuse policy. Instead, alcohol policy and drug policy have generally moved forward as parallel activities, involving different actors pursuing different agendas, and with science or research making, at best, a modest contribution in each of these two related arenas.

When the alcohol and illicit drugs stories are looked at together, it becomes clear just how difficult it is for policy makers to be governed by rationality when that rationality clashes with both 'conventional wisdom' and sectional interests of one kind or another. The conventional wisdom or cultural perspective on alcohol in Ireland appears to portray this substance as essentially benign; it is a familiar drug which has always been part of our everyday environment, so that epidemiological and public health arguments that it is a dangerous drug and that consumption levels and drinking patterns should be changed or regulated appear moralistic and out of touch with popular sentiment. It was argued in Chapter Two that, prior to the coming of the disease concept, Ireland could be considered to have had, in cultural and political terms, a balanced approach to alcohol and that at least some of this balance was lost by the relatively uncritical importation of a concept which was ideologically functional in the USA – its country of origin – but not obviously needed in Ireland. Be that as it may, the diffusion of the disease concept to Ireland contributed to the emergence of a new cultural perspective on alcohol, a perspective which was antithetical to public health in that it appeared to exaggerate the importance of individual predisposition while understating the negative attributes of alcohol.

On the other hand, illicit drugs, which are of more recent origin, have been conventionally portrayed and popularly accepted in Ireland as being unspeakably evil, so that it is acceptable and commonplace to describe public policy in this sphere in terms of a 'war on drugs'. Rational policy analysis suggests that neither supply reduction strategies nor demand reduction strategies have any real chance of making society drug-free, thereby winning the war on drugs. One only has to consider the failure of prison authorities to make Irish prisons drug free – and it should be made clear that Irish prison authorities are no more or less successful than their international counterparts generally – to realise how unrealistic it is to aim at insulating the country as a whole, so as to exclude illicit drugs. To some extent, drug use has become normalised, especially amongst young people, and demand-reduction strategies appear to offer relatively little hope of radically reversing or altering this situation. Instead, rational policy analysis tends to the view that it would be better to: (1) accept pragmatically that we must learn to live with some level of drug use; (2) avoid policy measures which may inflate harm; and (3) promote health through various forms of harm-reduction strategy. Such strategy would include primary preventive lifeskills education which might have universal application, as well as the methadone maintenance and needle exchange programmes discussed in Chapter Seven which might be more selectively targeted at sub-groups of established problem drug users. However, it also appears to be the case that to large sections of the general populace such harm-reduction strategies are immoral and quite unacceptable, and that, even if it is just to be a symbolic crusade, they remain devoted to the idea of a war on drugs and to the ideal of a drug-free society.

What has consistently emerged from the previous seven chapters is that, although there have been many actors involved in the policy process over the half century studied, ultimate decisions as to what Irish society will accept in this sphere are made by political leaders. Health care professionals, civil servants, church authorities, community activists, captains of industry and the media all contribute in important ways, but final decisions as to the shape of public policy on alcohol and illicit drugs are taken by elected politicians. As is to be expected in democratic societies, decisions of this type are largely dictated by politicians' judgements of what the electorate wishes or at least will tolerate. While it may seem obvious, what needs to be restated is that policy making is a political process rather than a rational or scientific process, and it is to be expected therefore that health policy will reflect what politicians judge to be electorally acceptable.

The epidemiological evidence and the general thrust of the public health perspective on alcohol suggests that, in the interests of health, Irish public policy on alcohol should become 'drier' and should utilise control strategies. These health promotional arguments for making alcohol consumption less easy for individual drinkers and for creating an environment in which alcohol is less normalised are presented in scientific terms. As Minister for Health, Michael Noonan was involved during 1996 in the launch of the long-awaited National Alcohol Policy. Although this policy document was quite vague and aspirational, and could certainly not be interpreted as being aggressively 'neo-prohibitionist', Mr Noonan was clearly uncomfortable with anything that smacked of paternalism in relation to alcohol. He told the press conference at the official launch of the policy that he was not planning 'to legislate for virtue' and that he favoured a situation in which citizens of Ireland would be provided with information but then left to 'make individual sovereign decisions in their own interest'.

Despite being Minister for Health, Mr Noonan had obviously decided that, whatever the scientific merits of the public health perspective, the Irish policy climate was not yet receptive to the radical alcohol-control strategies which this perspective entailed. Any lingering doubts which he might have had on this topic must have been banished by the controversy which attended the introduction of the Road Traffic Act, 1994 and the speedy softening of the new penalties for drunk driving contained in this legislation (see Chapter Four). The debacle which followed this attempt to make Irish roads safer demonstrated just how difficult it was to challenge cultural perceptions about alcohol or to operationalise the Ottawa Charter concept of 'healthy public policy' in this sphere. However, in the context of the two case-studies presented in this book, it is clear that Mr Noonan's remarks at the launch of the National Alcohol Policy are best understood as specific reassurance that he did not intend to engage in a radical drive to change Irish drinking habits, rather than as an expression of general philosophical beliefs which he planned to apply consistently as Minister for Health. If his libertarian views on alcohol consumption had been interpreted as also applying to the use of illicit drugs, there would certainly have been a political controversy greater even than that which arose from the introduction of the Road Traffic Act, 1994. Nobody interpreted his remarks in this way, however, or commented upon the double standard which was implicit therein: in relation to alcohol it was being suggested that Irish people should be left free to make their own choices, while in relation to currently illicit drugs a more paternalistic and prohibitionist regime remained unquestioned.

What emerges from an analysis of the two case studies is just how wide a gap there is between the rhetoric of health promotion and the political realities which have to be judged by elected leaders, particularly ministers. Politicians, rather than any of the other policy actors, are the ultimate judges of popular readiness to change, and it appeared to be their view that the Irish were not ready at the end of the period studied to accept what would in any event be a paradoxical change: that is, the simultaneous introduction of tougher and more paternalistic alcohol policies alongside more liberalised, or at least more pragmatic, drug policies – all in the name of health promotion.

Sociologists and others who have criticised health promotion, and particularly the concept of 'healthy public policy' on the grounds that it represents a new form of social control or 'health fascism', in which more and more aspects of human behaviour and social life are brought under the sway of medicine and health care, appear to have an exaggerated view of the power and influence of these latter institutions. Health promotionists in Ireland have not been particularly successful in persuading the populace that alcohol is more risky than it has been conventionally portrayed in recent times. Equally, of course, they have had only limited success in persuading the Irish public of the validity of harm-reduction models, which make it clear that illicit drugs are not as uniformly evil as they have been conventionally portrayed. In terms of policy co-ordination and public sector management, what is clear is that the Irish health sector has not succeeded in articulating a coherent health promotion strategy in relation to alcohol and illicit drugs to which other governmental sectors have given assent and active co-operation.

Community participation

As mentioned above and as discussed in greater detail in Chapter One, the concept of 'community participation' has been central to the wider health promotion project, featuring in all the key WHO texts, in Irish policy documents on this topic and in much of the secondary literature. In the Ottawa Charter, health promotion is defined as 'the process of enabling people to increase control over and improve their health'.[4] This is a democratic concept which challenges the power and control previously enjoyed, almost indeed monopolised, by health care professionals and health care authorities. In popular terminology, community participation in health promotion represents 'bottom-up' activity, and where communities fail to become spontaneously involved in such initiatives it is envisaged that the role of the 'experts' is to empower or facilitate such actions. However, the limitations of this concept have become evident throughout the detailed presentation of the two case studies in this book.

If the alcohol story is looked at first, it is apparent that over the course of the half-century studied no significant locally-based social movements of a health promotional nature emerged in the alcohol sphere. The only large-scale and enduring social movement in the alcohol field to make a definite impression in Ireland during this period was Alcoholics Anonymous (AA), which had come to Ireland, had adapted successfully to a policy climate which was very different to that of its country of origin, and had gone from strength to strength. As was pointed out in Chapter Two, AA as an organisation is solely concerned with providing help to individuals who wish to stop drinking, and is specifically precluded by its Traditions (that is, its written administrative charter) from taking a public stance on policy issues or becoming involved in lobbying for any policy or form of service provision. This is not to detract in any way from the value of AA for individual problem drinkers, but merely to make the point that it is not concerned with problem prevention in any broad health promotional sense. As discussed in Chapters Two, Three and Four, AA was one element in the wider 'disease concept', an individualistic concept which purported to integrate drinking problems into a conventional biomedical framework and which was largely antithetical to health promotion.

For much of the period studied, but particularly in the late 1950s and throughout the 1960s, the disease concept was promoted in Ireland in a modernist way as representing a new scientific and non-moralistic approach to drinking problems; in this view, drinking problems could be primarily explained in terms of the individual deficits or predispositions of a minority of drinkers, with little responsibility being attributed to alcohol itself. The Department of Health played no role in the initial introduction of the disease concept to Ireland but did eventually adopt this approach, the high point of which was its espousal of and financial support for the Irish National Council on Alcoholism (INCA) in the early 1970s. By the time the Department of Health began to move tentatively towards its exploration of the public health perspective in the late 1970s, important changes had taken place in Irish drinking practices: there had been a generalised decline in temperance sentiment and an accompanying normalisation of alcohol, with particular increases in numbers of women drinkers and young drinkers. However, even following the establishment of the Health Promotion Unit in the Department of Health in 1988 and the decision to formulate a national alcohol policy, no significant initiatives to empower local or community-based alcohol prevention programmes emanated from the Department of Health. The policy-making process favoured by the Health Promotion Unit in its development of the national alcohol policy was not of the *organisational networking* style; even the working group which ostensibly had the responsibility of drafting this policy was excluded by the HPU from anything but the most superficial participation in the policy process. This obviously did not bode well for future networking and collaboration with local groups on alcohol issues.

In the completed text *National Alcohol Policy – Ireland* (1996) there is just a half-page section which deals with community initiatives, starting with the declaration that: 'Community action has the potential to be a powerful influence for both social and environment-directed interventions'. However, the remainder of this section is vague and unconvincing on this topic, citing just two Irish examples of 'best practice' in this sphere: the first of these refers to a Southern Health Board training programme in health education for professionals and volunteers who work with community groups, while the second describes parental initiatives to organise alcohol-free discos for teenagers in various parts of the country. The 'Action Plan' of this policy document is equally vague and brief on this theme, promising merely that the Department of Health will 'Support community initiatives which promote the National Alcohol Policy' and then referring in broad terms to youth work programmes.

National Alcohol Policy – Ireland makes brief reference to international research on the development of community prevention programmes, some of which have taken place in countries (such as Finland and Sweden) where the policy climate is more favourable to temperance than is the case in Ireland. However, no detailed discussion of these programmes is offered nor, as stated above, is there any strategy outlined for developing similar programmes in Ireland. It has to be concluded, therefore, that there is no evidence of the spontaneous emergence of any significant community initiatives aimed at the prevention of alcohol-related problems in Ireland; neither does it appear that the Health Promotion Unit, as it is currently structured, has the will or the capacity to mobilise or empower effective community initiatives. The reality is that, in most instances, communal celebrations in Ireland have alcohol consumption as a central element and may indeed be sponsored by the drinks industry; this is a reality which is far from the rhetoric of health promotion and community participation.

When the focus is switched to community participation in preventing or responding to problems associated with the use of illicit drugs, a different but equally complex set of questions is raised about the realisation of health promotional ideals. During the period described as the 'opiate epidemic' (1980-1985) there was an unprecedented rise in community development activities focused on heroin use in those areas of Dublin with the highest prevalence of such problems. In contrast to the situation which prevailed in relation to alcohol, there was no shortage of bottom-up initiatives aimed both at primary prevention and at treatment and rehabilitation of existing problems. Individually and collectively, these community responses to heroin could be seen as ideal types of health promotion activity: they involved local residents and locally-based primary health and social service personnel working collaboratively to deal with the heroin problems at local community level. The statutory health authorities (specifically the Eastern Health Board and the National Drug Advisory and Treatment Centre) rather than welcoming community participation of this kind and seeking to work in partnership with it, appeared to regard it as impertinent and demonstrated considerable antipathy towards the vision of those involved in community responses to heroin problems. The statutory health service response was based on a traditional biomedical model which viewed heroin addicts as individual 'patients' and took little stock of environmental factors; it was assumed within this traditional framework that treatment of addicts was best delivered by health care experts, preferably in centralised and specialist services. Even when the Eastern Health Board began to become more directly involved in the provision of addiction counselling within its Community Care services, this type of service provision was of a traditional – albeit decentralised – clinical style, provided by 'experts', aimed at individuals, and with little or no reference to community participation.

In summary, it can be said that the health promotional perspective of community activists who worked to develop local responses to heroin problems was not welcomed by the health authorities, and that the attitude of these authorities to the burgeoning community response to drugs was not one of partnership and support but rather one of considerable antipathy. Even as late as 1995, the first attempt at formal partnership between the Eastern Health Board and a local drug agency – the Ballymun Youth Action Project – had collapsed in acrimony and disarray, and it was only in 1996 that the First Report of the Ministerial Task Force on Measures to Reduce the Demand for Drugs established the structure of the Local Drugs Task Force to facilitate partnerships at community level.

This delay in setting up community-based responses, consisting of the collaboration of the statutory health authorities and local groupings, was perhaps predictable. Government in Ireland has tended to be highly centralised, with an underdeveloped local government sector, so it is not surprising that the concept of community care in the Irish health system has generally been interpreted by health service administrators as referring to the provision of non-institutional services rather than to the development of radical participative structures at local level. Furthermore, health care professionals have generally been socialised within traditional education and training systems, which emphasise their technical expertise and which do not readily predispose them to power-sharing with lay people.

It would be misleading, however, to convey the impression that local participation in the response to heroin or other serious drug problems invariably reflects a communal consensus of a welfare type, a consensus which is invariably benign towards drug users and is automatically superior to service provision by professionals. Some community activism took the form of aggressive rejection of both drug *dealers* and drug *users*, categories which frequently overlap and sometimes are effectively indistinguishable in local drug scenes. Informal community policing, which appears on the face of it to be a liberal and worthwhile venture, can quickly turn into aggressive vigilante activity, and certainly there were occasions when unofficial evictions or opposition to proposed local treatment services suggested that activists, while protecting their communities, were reinforcing and perpetuating the social exclusion of drug users. Similarly, community groups when they were consulted on this topic, did not always collaborate with the health authorities in the creation of locally-based treatment services, but sometimes – and this was increasingly the norm as methadone programmes became commonplace – were bitterly opposed to the siting of services and facilities in their neighbourhoods. It could be argued that had the statutory authorities been quicker to form partnerships with community groups, this might have led to a less aggressive form of community activism. It could equally be argued that the notion of community participation in health promotion has been propounded uncritically and superficially, without due recognition of its negative potential. In his 1982 minority report to the Barclay Report on community social work in Britain, Robert Pinker suggested that: 'It is one of the stubbornly persistent illusions in social policy studies that eventually the concept of community – as a basis of shared values – will resolve all our policy dilemmas'.[5] Later in this report, Pinker argued explicitly that local or community-based services were not necessarily welcomed by their recipients: specifically, he concluded that in the history of British social policy it was the nineteenth-century Poor Law which was the most localised and intimate form of service provision, and that it 'was just this distinctive quality of parochial social service that added a uniquely hurtful dimension to the experience of stigma among the recipients of poor relief'.[6]

In Britain there has been little detailed study to date of local partnership approaches to the management of drug problems, but in a review of British drug policy MacGregor commented in passing on the negative potential of such activity; referring back to the tradition of the Poor Law, she speculated that drug users could become 'a new stratum of vagrants excluded from each parish's social provision ...'.[7] While it falls just outside the timeframe for the present study, it should be noted that the enactment in Ireland of the Housing (Miscellaneous Provisions) Act, 1997, ostensibly aimed at fostering community participation in 'estate management' and facilitating the eviction of 'anti-social' tenants, is another example of a policy development which may have the unintended consequence of scapegoating and excluding drug users and their families from the neighbourhoods in which they live.

In conclusion, it seems clear from this study of Irish alcohol and drug policy in the second half of the twentieth century that the notion of community participation in health promotion is a great deal more complex and contentious than is suggested in formal aspirational policy statements on this topic. It also seems clear that if health promotion is to move beyond rhetoric in this area of community participation, it must acknowledge and grapple with the tensions and ambiguities identified here.

Individual lifestyles

To members of the public with just a passing acquaintance with health promotion, it may be that its very essence consists of educational messages advising them that their health status is largely determined by their 'lifestyles' and urging them accordingly to cultivate healthy lifestyles. However, it was made clear in Chapter One that health promotion philosophy as developed and enunciated by WHO was intended to incorporate both *individualistic* and *communitarian/collectivist* approaches to health, and that policy which consisted solely of individualistic strategies could not really be regarded as coming under the rubric of health promotion. Individualism as a philosophy is usually associated with traditional conservative or New Right politics and is regarded as antithetical to public health. It is commonly assumed that individualism is popular with such political groupings because it does not question or disturb existing economic arrangements or call for any radical restructuring of society in the interests of social justice or equity. The data presented in this study also suggest, however, that individualistic health promotion of this kind – when analysed in its own right and leaving aside these major socio-economic issues – can throw up a range of technical and moral complications.

In relation to alcohol, it has proven difficult for health educators to come up with any clear message with which to replace the comforting idea that personal levels of consumption are unimportant for most drinkers who are not 'alcoholic'. By 1996, when the National Alcohol Policy was eventually published, the validity and practical utility of 'sensible' or 'safe' drinking guidelines presented in terms of 'units' of alcohol – which had been popular for the previous decade – had been questioned to such an extent that they were simply dropped in this country. There is, in absolute terms, no such thing as a 'safe' drinking level: alcohol consumption carries risk regardless of dosage, although this risk is clearly influenced by dosage/consumption level, as it is by pattern and by a host of other individual and contextual factors. What appeared to be emerging, therefore, from this view of risk was that educational messages should be aimed at specific groups, such as drivers, students or pregnant women rather than at an undifferentiated public. The fact that moderate alcohol consumption appears to confer health benefit also complicates the task of health educators, and perhaps the overall conclusion one might reach from a close reading of this part of the National Alcohol Policy was that the Department of Health had by now developed a keen sense of how contentious this topic could be and was committed, above all else, to avoiding trouble.

In overall terms, the findings of this study confirm that, as was the case with other elements of health promotion, the implementation of programmes aimed at fostering healthy lifestyles is considerably more difficult than is suggested by the relatively superficial rhetoric of national and international policy documents on this topic.

Treatment in a reoriented health service?

The health promotional aspiration to a 'reoriented health service', one in which prevention of illness is given priority over curative functions and in which access to primary health care is seen as more important than the creation of specialist services, is the last specific element of the Ottawa Charter to be considered here. The term 'primary health care' is somewhat ambiguous in developed countries, but generally it is taken to refer above all else to the roles and functions of general medical practitioners, in association with other locally-based non-specialists in the paramedical field. There are a number of obvious practical problems which militate against the development of a major health-promoting role by GPs, and some of these will now be looked at in the context of health service responses to drug and alcohol problems.

First of all, as discussed in Chapter One, health promotion as a concept did not originate within the medical profession, and the professional socialisation of doctors has tended to continue with its emphasis on curative functions within a traditional biomedical model. Secondly, it is also important to note that within the Irish healthcare scene, as in many countries, GPs are independent professionals rather than health service employees and, as such, may not be especially familiar with or well-disposed towards official pronouncements about health promotion. Finally, general medical practice is based upon seeing large numbers of patients for relatively brief consultations, and the complex psychosocial issues raised by problem drinkers and problem drug users may not be readily managed within this context.

Chapter Four, which dealt with the formulation of the National Alcohol Policy, concluded that by and large no reorientation of the health service had taken place or seemed imminent in relation to alcohol. The creation of community-based alcoholism treatment programmes did not automatically lead to substantial reductions in hospital admissions for such problems; on the contrary, in-patient admissions for drinking problems remained stubbornly high, although length of stay for such admissions did shorten. No specific strategy for changing the attitudes or practices of GPs with regard to alcohol consumption and related problems was devised, and referral to specialist services – either the in-patient mental health system or the new community alcoholism services – appeared to be the norm. Furthermore, it seemed as though the disease concept had become culturally integrated into the Irish psyche to the extent that the public had now come to expect that alcoholism *should* be treated in in-patient settings and also to view community-based services as technically inferior or second-best. If, as was suggested explicitly in Chapter Three, there were two conflicting paradigms – the disease concept and the public health or health promotional perspective on alcohol – then it would have to be concluded that, both in terms of professional practice and popular expectation, the disease concept was an easy winner.

The response of the Irish healthcare system to illicit drug use and its related problems, when viewed in terms of a 'reoriented' service, was found to be different though equally problematic. For most of the period studied, Irish healthcare policy was based on an implicit assumption that illicit drug users were a deviant and devious group, quite unsuited to primary healthcare and best treated in specialist settings away from 'normal' patients. One element of this philosophy was the view that GPs who became clinically involved with drug users might be cajoled or coerced into inappropriate prescribing, thus perpetuating rather than resolving the problem of dependency. Those few GPs who had participated energetically and conscientiously in bottom-up community programmes during the era of the 'opiate epidemic', as described in Chapter Six, were neither thanked nor encouraged for taking this initiative, and it was only in the late 1980s – when the relationship between needle-sharing and HIV transmission amongst injecting drug users became apparent – that official policy began to swing towards the view that family doctors had a role to play in the management of drug problems.

As detailed in Chapter Seven, the task of involving GPs in this activity, and in particular the task of institutionalising methadone prescribing by GPs, was a difficult and complex one which was tackled in a relatively covert way through small policy-making networks co-ordinated by the Department of Health. By 1996, however, significant progress had been made on the establishment of a formalised system or protocol which promised to normalise methadone prescribing by making it more accessible through general medical practice, while at the same time setting in place controls and safeguards which were intended to prevent malpractice in this area and avoid leakage of methadone into the black market. There is, however, no getting away from the contentious nature of methadone maintenance, especially when it is normalised within general medical practice. To those who favour it, the creation of a GP's methadone protocol represents a humane and pragmatic policy development which is effective and evidence-based; to its opponents, such a protocol simply facilitates the cynical use of medical technology for social-control purposes. It would appear, however, that because of the urgency of the public health situation created by HIV/AIDS and the perceived necessity to introduce harm-reduction measures, more progress was made on reorienting the health service in relation to illicit drugs than was the case with alcohol.

Ultimately, perhaps all that can be concluded is that abstract statements about reorienting health services and maximising the role of primary healthcare systems provide relatively little practical guidance for health policy makers. Some pragmatic successes have been achieved in relation to the management of illicit drug problems by primary healthcare systems, despite the cultural ambivalence and value conflicts which characterise the harm reduction field, but as yet little progress has been made in relation to alcohol problems.

Policy making for health promotion

As pointed out earlier in this chapter, advocates of health promotion have been more forthright in setting out their aims and objectives than in providing detailed accounts of *how* these aims and objectives might be achieved. While academic authors have attempted to look in detail at the policy-making process and at the utility of various models of policy-making, the emphasis in official policy documents (particularly the Irish health policy documents referred to throughout this book) has been almost entirely on the statement of aims and objectives. The three models of policy co-ordination outlined by Harrison and Tether (1987) and discussed in Chapter One – the *rational-comprehensive, partisan mutual adjustment* and *organisational networks* models – have, by and large, been useful for analytic purposes. It may be said by way of generalised concluding comment that the policy events described in this book have usually been discussed and framed in terms of rationality (the first model), implemented incrementally and with much compromise (in accordance with the second model), but have shown most promise in health promotional terms when they have occasionally involved organisational networking (the third model). This conclusion will now be discussed in some detail.

The early Irish policy documents which deal with health promotion tended to be implicitly based upon rationalistic assumptions. Increasingly, however, they have made explicit use of a rational or *managerialist* approach to health policy and service provision, largely consisting of the establishment of national goals and targets the achievement of which, it is suggested, would promote the health of the nation. This managerialist approach is exemplified in the 1995 document *A Health Promotion Strategy: Making the healthier choice the easier choice* which was referred to earlier in this chapter. Goal and target setting of this kind is based on an economic rationalism which does not, in the main, acknowledge the complexities and difficulties of health promotion, discussed initially in Chapter One of this study and then illustrated in detail in the subsequent eight chapters. There is no reason to conclude, on the basis of the material presented in this book, that such mechanistic goal and target setting has anything to contribute to health promotion in relation to alcohol and drugs; and academic policy analysis is generally sceptical of its appropriateness and value in an arena characterised by philosophical ambiguity, political conflict and competing economic interests.

The health-promoting structures which were established in Ireland in the late 1980s (and which were discussed in Chapters One and Four) could not generally be deemed to have been a success in creating and sustaining a dynamic policy process. The Cabinet sub-committee on health promotion which was at the top of the structural pyramid appears not to have functioned at all; referring to this element of the total structure, Cecily Kelleher (Professor of Health Promotion at University College Galway) has written cryptically: 'A new cabinet sub-committee for health promotion was formed comprising relevant ministries influencing health status, though in fact this group never met in plenary'.[8] It seems reasonable to infer from this that high-level political commitment to the concept of health promotion was lacking. The findings of this study generally suggest that there is no consistent political commitment to the application of health promotion concepts to alcohol policy, but rather that politicians selectively pursue or support particular initiatives when they deem these initiatives to have popular support. However, it has also been shown that on those occasions when politicians of at least Minister of State level became personally involved in the formulation of policy on illicit drugs, this accelerated the policy-making process and gave it a new impetus. (In this context, one of the more important outcomes of the Rabbitte Report of 1996 was the creation of new policy and management structures for illicit drug problems, including the establishment of a Cabinet committee on drugs.) In the absence of sustained high-level political commitment to health promotion, a great deal depended upon two other elements of the structure – the Advisory Council on Health Promotion and the Health Promotion Unit. However, on the evidence of their performance in formulating a national alcohol policy, neither of these structures was effective in realising health promotional ideals. The failure of these structures is acknowledged in *A Health Promotion Strategy: Making the healthier choice the easier choice* where, without detailed or critical analysis, it is concluded that: 'Experience would suggest, however, that there are certain shortcomings – largely of a practical nature – associated with those arrangements'. This report then proposed to replace the *Advisory Council on Health Promotion* with a new *National Consultative Committee on Health Promotion,* although in the absence of detailed supporting argument or critical analysis it was difficult to see how this innovation involved anything other than a change of name.

The Health Promotion Unit itself, judged by its performance in relation to the drafting and implementation of the national alcohol policy, must also be deemed to have been a disappointment. Much was expected of the HPU following the creation of the so-called health promotion structures in 1988, yet little or no explicit discussion took place as to how it should function or how the culture of this sub-unit of a much larger department should differ from the culture of the parent department in its pursuit of its own specific goals. The rational tone of official pronouncements on the national alcohol policy gave no hint of the cultural and economic conflicts which characterised this domain, and which became immediately apparent to the HPU. Its management of this policy-making task could be deemed to have been a success only in that a policy document was eventually produced, and without any major public controversy such as that which surrounded the Health Education Bureau's lifeskills programme. It may be deemed a failure, however, in that it did not create or sustain an organisational network of like-minded people who shared a serious commitment to furthering the health promotion agenda on alcohol. The HPU opted not to see its task in terms of a policy process which would be best advanced by forming external alliances, but instead fell back on the traditional central government department tactic of controlling the situation, defusing potential conflict and being satisfied with minor gains. This is not to say that all sections of the Department of Health invariably follow this model of policy making, and it was noted in Chapter Seven that, in response to the public health crisis which arose in relation to needle-sharing amongst intravenous drug users, an organisational networks approach was adopted and applied – with considerable skill and success – to the expansion of methadone maintenance treatment services.

To conclude on a positive note, by the end of the study period the concept of organisational networks in public sector management in Ireland had become popular in the context of the wider *Strategic Management Initiative,* and it was explicitly recognised that important public policy goals could only be achieved through partnership arrangements between different sectors of Government, as well as the collaboration of non-governmental agencies. It was argued in Chapter Seven that the work of the ministerial group which led to the publication of the so-called *Rabbitte Report,* although not based in the Department of Health, had done more to advance health promotion in the illicit drugs field than any initiative previously emanating from Health. The *National Drugs Strategy Team* which resulted from this report may be seen as a somewhat formalised version of the organisational networks discussed in Harrison and Tether (1987), and it too remained outside Health, although it had a senior civil servant from Health as a team-member. While it is too early to form any definitive judgement on the effectiveness of this National Drugs Strategy Team, it is clear that it represents a new approach to policy making and implementation in relation to illicit drugs, and it is interesting to consider whether a similar body could ever be established in the alcohol field.

Health promotion – a realistic proposition?

In purely abstract terms, health promotion makes sense: the health of individuals and of whole societies is dependent upon a great deal more than the effectiveness of curative treatment systems, and it would appear self-evidently good that illnesses should be prevented and positive health fostered. However, the detailed application of the Ottawa Charter to Irish drug and alcohol policy, which has made up the bulk of this book and which has been reviewed in this chapter, reveals a myriad of difficulties and complexities which characterise health promotion. In everyday life there are countless instances where behavioural choices are based upon immediate gratification or laziness rather than health: people don't always wear their seatbelts on short car journeys, they don't always floss or brush their teeth thoroughly if they are tired, or they sit down and look at television for the night when the healthy alternative would be to go for a walk. Health is often taken for granted, and in the pursuit of other understandable goals – money or pleasure, for instance – the hope is that illness can be avoided or that the healthcare system will cure such illnesses as do occur.

Ultimately, what this detailed study of alcohol, illicit drugs and health promotion suggests is that there is a big gap between the ambitious rhetoric of health promotionists and the realities of human behaviour and public policy. As things currently stand, health promotion is not a realistic proposition, but merely a pious aspiration. The first step to closing this gap would seem to involve acknowledging its existence. The Ottawa Charter can still serve as a framework for the realisation of health promotion ideals, but it would seem clear that it can only succeed when policy makers move from the level of rhetoric to a more pragmatic style of health strategy which takes full account of the difficulties identified here.

NOTES

1. See, for example, I. Illich, *Limits to Medicine: Medical Nemesis.* (London: Marion Boyars, 1977).
2. As an example of this use of the phrase by advocates of health promotion see J. Ashton and H. Seymour, *The New Public Health: The Liverpool Experience.* (Milton Keynes: Open University Press, 1988); for a more critical sociological exploration of this concept see A. Petersen and D. Lupton, *The New Public Health: health and self in the age of risk.* (London: Sage Publications, 1996).
3. See *A Health Promotion Strategy: Making the healthier choice the easier choice.* (Dublin: Department of Health, 1995).
4. *Ottawa Charter for Health Promotion.* (Geneva: WHO, 1986), p.1.
5. R. Pinker, 'An alternative view' in *Social Workers: Their Role and Task.* (London: Bedford Square Press, 1982), p.241.
6. Ibid., p. 245.
7. S. MacGregor, 'Medicine, Custom or Moral Fibre: Policy Responses to Drug Misuse' in N. South (ed.), *Drugs: Cultures, Controls and Everyday Life.* (London: Sage, 1999), p.83.
8. C. Kelleher, 'Promoting Health', in J. Robins (ed.), *Reflections on Health: Commemorating Fifty Years of the Department of Health 1947-1997.* (Dublin: Institute of Public Administration, 1977), p.37.

Bibliography

AA Member, 'Rehabilitating the Alcoholic', *The Furrow* (May 1956), pp 276-284.

A Dublin Member of AA, 'Vatican and Alcoholics Anonymous', in 'News and Views', *The Furrow* (March, 1972), p. 182.

Advisory Committee on Drug Dependence, *Cannabis.* (London: Her Majesty's Stationery Office, 1968).

Advisory Council on the Misuse of Drugs, *Treatment and Rehabilitation.* (London: Her Majesty's Stationery Office, 1982).

Advisory Council on the Misuse of Drugs, *AIDS and Drug Misuse (Part 1).* (London: Her Majesty's Stationery Office, 1988).

A Framework for Partnership: Enriching Strategic Consensus through Participation. (Dublin: National Economic and Social Forum, 1997).

A Health Promotion Strategy: Making the Healthier Choice the Easier Choice. (Dublin: Department of Health, 1995).

Alcoholics Anonymous, *Alcoholics Anonymous* (First edition). (New York, AA World Publishing, 1939).

Alcoholics Anonymous, *Twelve Steps and Twelve Traditions.* (New York, AA Publishing, 1952).

Alcoholics Anonymous in Ireland 1946-1986: A souvenir booklet to commemorate forty years of AA in Ireland. (Dublin: AA General Service Conference of Ireland, 1986).

A Member, 'Alcoholics Anonymous', *The Furrow* (November 1953), pp 638-647.

Anderson, D., *Perspectives on Treatment: The Minnesota Experience.* (Center City, Minnesota: Hazelden, 1981).

⌐ Anderson, D. (ed.), *Drinking to Your Health: The Allegations and the Evidence.* (London: Social Affairs Unit, 1989).

Anderson, R. 'Critique of Today Tonight's Programme on Alcoholism, 20th December 1982', *Irish Social Worker,* 2, (1983), p. 16.

Ashton, J. and Seymour, H., *The New Public Health: The Liverpool Experience.* (Milton Keynes: Open University Press, 1988).

A Victim, 'Alcoholism', *The Furrow* (March 1953), pp 139-146.

Bachrach, P. and Baratz,M., 'Decisions and Nondecisions: An Analytical Framework', *American Political Science Review,* 57 (1963), pp 632-642.

Bachrach, P. and Baratz, M., *Power and Poverty: Theory and Practice.* (Oxford University Press, 1970).

Bacon, S., 'Sociology and the Problems of Alcohol: Foundations for a Sociologic Study of Drinking Behaviour', *Quarterly Journal of Studies on Alcohol ,* 4 (1943), pp 402-412.

Bacon, S., 'Discussion: Social Science' in Keller, M. (ed.), *Journal of Studies on Alcohol (Supplement 8),* (1979), pp 289-321.

⌐ Baggot, R., *Alcohol, Politics and Social Policy.* (Aldershot: Gower, 1990).

Baggot, R., 'Alcohol, Politics and Social Policy', *Journal of Social Policy,* 15 (1987), pp 467-488.

Barrington, R., *Health, Medicine and Politics in Ireland 1900-1970.* (Dublin: Institute of Public Administration, 1987).

Barrington, T., 'Whatever Happened to Irish Government? *Administration,* 30 (1982), pp 89-112.

Baum, F. and Saunders, D., 'Can health promotion and primary health care achieve Health for All without a return to their more radical agenda?', *Health Promotion International,* 10 (1995), pp 149-160.

Beauchamp, D., *Beyond Alcoholism: Alcohol and Public Health Policy.* (Philadelphia: Temple University Press, 1980).

Becker, H., *Outsiders: Studies in the Sociology of Deviance.* (New York: The Free Press, 1963).

Bennet, D., 'Are They Always Right? Investigation and proof in a citizen anti-heroin movement', in Tomlinson, M., Varley, T. and McCullagh, C. (eds), *Whose Law and Order? Aspects of crime and social control in Irish society.* (Sociological Association of Ireland, 1988), pp 21-40.

Bowden, M., *Rialto Community Drug Team.* (Dublin: Rialto Community Drug Team, 1996).

Boyle, R., *The Management of Cross-Cutting Issues.* (Dublin: Institute of Public Administration, 1999).

Bratter, T., Bratter, E. and Heinberg, J., 'Uses and Abuses of Power and Authority Within the American Self-Help Residential Therapeutic Community', in De Leon, G. and Ziegenfuss, J. (eds), *Therapeutic Communities for Addictions: Readings in Theory, Research and Practice.* (Springfield Illinois: Charles C. Thomas, 1986), pp 191-207.

Brown, P., 'Popular epidemiology: community response to toxic-waste induced disease in Woburn, Massachusetts', *Science, Technology and Human Values,* 12 (1987), pp 78-85.

Bruun, K., Pan, L. and Rexed, I., *The Gentlemen's Club: International Control of Drugs and Alcohol.* (University of Chicago Press, 1975).

Bruun, K. et al, *Alcohol Control Policies in Public Health Perspective.* (Helsinki: Finnish Foundation for Alcohol Studies, 1975).

Building on Reality 1984-1987. (Dublin: Stationery Office, 1984).

Bunton, R., Nettleton, S., and Burrows, R. (eds), *The Sociology of Health Promotion: Critical Analyses of Consumption, Lifestyle and Risk.* (London: Routledge, 1995).

Butler, S., 'Drug Problems and Drug Policies in Ireland: A Quarter of a Century Reviewed', *Administration,* 39 (1991), pp 210-233.

Butler, S., 'Alcohol and Drug Education in Ireland: Aims, Methods and Difficulties', *Oideas,* 42 (1994), pp 125-140.

Butler, S. and Woods, M., 'Drugs, HIV and Ireland: Responses to Women in Dublin', in Dorn, N., Henderson, S. and South, N. (eds), *AIDS: Women, Drugs and Social Care.* (London: Falmer Press, 1992), pp 51-69.

Byrne, D. et al, 'Strategic Management in the Irish Civil Service: A Review Drawing on New Zealand and Australia', *Administration,* 43 (Special Issue, No. 2, 1995).

Cahalan, D., *Problem Drinkers.* (San Francisco: Jossey Bass, 1970).

Cahalan, D. and Room, R., *Problem Drinking Among American Men.* (New Brunswick, New Jersey: Rutgers Centre of Alcohol Studies, 1974).

Cahalan, D., *Understanding America's Drinking Problems: How to Combat the Hazards of Alcohol.* (San Francisco: Jossey-Bass, 1987).

'Care of the Drug Addict' (Editorial), *Journal of the Irish Medical Association,* 64 (1971), p. 148.

Charleton, P., 'Drugs and Crime – Making the Connection: A Discussion', *Irish Criminal Law Journal,* 5 (1995), pp 220-240.

Christie, N. and Bruun, K., 'Alcohol Problems: The Conceptual Framework' in Keller, M. and Coffey, T. (eds), *Proceedings of the 28th International Congress on Alcohol and Alcoholism.* (Highland Park, New Jersey: Hillouse Press, 1969).

Chubb, B., *The Government and Politics of Ireland* (2nd ed.), (London: Longman, 1982).

Clare, A., *Psychiatry in Dissent: Controversial Issues in Thought and Practice.* (London: Tavistock, 1976).

Comberton, J., *Drugs and Young People.* (Dublin: Ward River Press, 1982).

Comberton, P., 'Drug Addiction and AIDS', *Irish Social Worker,* 8 (1), (1989), pp 9-10.

Conniffe, D. and McCoy, D., *Alcohol Use in Ireland: The Economic and Social Implications.* (Dublin: Economic and Social Research Institute, 1992).

Connolly, J., *Family Doctors and Alcoholism.* (Unpublished Masters in Community Education Thesis, St Patrick's College, Maynooth, 1994).

'Conversation with Vincent Dole', *Addiction,* 89 (1994), pp 23-29.

Cooney, J., 'Alcoholism and Addiction in General Practice', *Irish Medical Journal,* 53 (1963), pp 53-55.

Cooney, J., 'Alcoholism and the Psychiatrist', *Journal of the Irish Medical Association,* 73 (1980), pp 104-111.

Cooney, J., *Under the Weather: Alcoholism and Alcohol Abuse – How to Cope.* (Dublin: Gill and Macmillan, 1991).

Cooney, J., *John Charles McQuaid: Ruler of Catholic Ireland.* (Dublin: O'Brien Press, 1999).

Courtwright, D., 'The prepared mind: Marie Nyswander, methadone maintenance and the metabolic theory of addiction', *Addiction* 92, (1997), pp 257-265.

Cronin, J., 'The Question of Needle Exchange', *Irish Social Worker,* 8(1), (1989), pp 11-12.

Cullen, B., *Community and Drugs: A case study in community conflict in the inner city of Dublin.* (Unpublished M.Litt. thesis, Trinity College Dublin, 1992).

Cullen, B., 'Community Action in the Eighties: A Case Study', in *Community Work in Ireland: Trends in the 80s, Options for the 90s.* (Dublin: Combat Poverty Agency, 1990), pp 271-294.

Davies, P., 'Motivation, Responsibility and Sickness in the Psychiatric Treatment of Alcoholism', *British Journal of Psychiatry,* 134 (1979), pp 447-451.

Davies, P. and Walsh, D., *Alcohol Problems and Alcohol Control in Europe.* (London: Croom Helm, 1983).

Dean, G., Bradshaw, J. and Lavelle, P., *Drug Misuse in Dublin 1982-1983: Investigation in a North Central Dublin Area and in Galway, Sligo and Cork.* (Dublin: Medico-Social Research Board, 1983).

De Leon, G. and Schwartz, S., 'Therapeutic Communities: What Are the Retention Rates?', *American Journal of Drug and Alcohol Abuse,* 10 (1984), pp 267-284.

Delivering Better Government: Second Report to Government of the Co-ordinating Group of Secretaries. (Dublin: Stationery Office, 1996).

Des Jarlais, D. et al, 'HIV Incidence Among Injecting Drug Users in New York City Syringe Exchange Programmes', *The Lancet,* 348 (1996), pp 987-991.

Dorn, N. and Murji, K., *Drug Prevention: A Review of the English Language Literature.* (London: Institute for the Study of Drug Dependence, 1992).

Douglas, M., *Risk and Blame: Essays in Cultural Theory.* (London: Routledge, 1992).

Edwards, G., 'Addiction: A Challenge to Society', *New Society* (October 25, 1984).

Edwards, G., 'What Drives British Drug Policy?', *British Journal of Addiction,* 84 (1989), pp 219 -223.

Edwards, G., Keller, M., Moser, J. and Room, R., *Alcohol-Related Disabilities.* (WHO Offset Publications Number 320), (Geneva: World Health Organisation, 1977).

Edwards, G. et al, *Alcohol Policy and the Public Good.* (Oxford University Press, 1994).

Engelsman, E., 'Dutch Policy on the Management of Drug-Related Problems', *British Journal of Addiction,* 84 (1989), pp 211-218.

European Monitoring Centre for Drugs and Drug Addiction, *1996 Annual Report on the State of the Drugs Problem in the European Union.* (Lisbon: European Monitoring Centre for Drugs and Drug Addiction, 1997).

Feeney, J., *John Charles McQuaid: the man and the mask.* (Cork: Mercier Press, 1974).

Ferriter, D., *A Nation of Extremes: The Pioneers in Twentieth-Century Ireland.* (Dublin: Irish Academic Press, 1999).

Finnane, M., *Insanity and the Insane in Post-Famine Ireland.* (London: Croom Helm, 1981).

First Annual Report of the National Co-ordinating Committee on Drug Abuse. (Dublin: Stationery Office, 1986).

First Report of the Ministerial Task Force on Measures to Reduce the Demand for Drugs. (Dublin: Department of the Taoiseach, 1996).

FitzGerald, J., Quinn, T., Whelan, B. and Williams, J., *An Analysis of Cross-Border Shopping.* (Dublin: Economic and Social Research Institute, 1988).

Flynn, S. and Yeates, P., *Smack: The Criminal Drugs Racket in Ireland.* (Dublin: Gill and Macmillan, 1985).

Ford, J., 'The Priest's Role in Alcohol Problems', *The Furrow* (May 1960), pp 285-300.

Forrestal, C., *Evaluation Report on Ballymun Community Drug Team.* (Dublin: Community Action Network, 1996).

Freedman, D., Shattock, A., Stuart, J. and McLaughlin, H., 'Acquired immunodeficiency syndrome', *Irish Medical Journal,* 82 (1989), pp 135-138.

Garvin, T., *1922: The Birth of Irish Democracy.* (Dublin: Gill and Macmillan, 1996).

Ghodse, H., 'International Policies on Addiction: Strategy development and cooperation', *British Journal of Psychiatry,* 166 (1995), pp 14-18.

Giesbrecht, N., *Consequences of Drinking: Trends in Alcohol Problem Statistics in Seven Countries.* (Toronto: Addiction Research Foundation, 1983).

Glanz, A., 'The fall and rise of the general practitioner' in Strang, J. and Gossop, M. (eds), *Heroin Addiction and Drug Policy: The British System.* (Oxford University Press, 1994), pp 151-166.

Government Strategy to Prevent Drug Misuse. (Dublin: Department of Health, 1991).

Green Paper on Mental Health. (Dublin: Stationery Office, 1992).

Guldan, G., 'Obstacles to Community Health Promotion, *Social Science and Medicine,* 42 (1996), pp 689-695.

Gusfield, J., 'Prohibition: The Impact of Poltical Utopianism' in Braeman, J. et al (eds), *Change and Continuity in Twentieth-Century America.* (Columbus: Ohio State University Press, 1968).

Gusfield, J., *Symbolic Crusade: Status, Politics and the American Temperance Movement* (2nd ed.). (Urbana: University of Illinois Press, 1986).

Halleck, S., 'The great drug education hoax', *The Progressive ,* 34 (1970), pp. 1-7, cited in Swisher, J., 'Addiction Prevention – Future Directions', *Proceedings of the Health Education Bureau Conference: Education Against Addiction,* 1979, p. 68.

Ham, C. and Hill, M., *The Policy Process in the Modern Capitalist State* (2nd ed.). (Brighton: Wheatsheaf Books, 1993).

Harrison, L. and Tether, P., 'The Co-ordination of UK Policy on Alcohol and Tobacco: The significance of organisational networks', *Policy and Politics,* 15 (1987), pp 77-90.

Health: The Wider Dimensions – A Consultative Statement on Health Policy. (Dublin: Department of Health, 1986).

Heath, D., 'Policies, Politics and Pseudo-science: A cautionary tale about alcohol controls', in Anderson, D., *Drinking to Your Health: The allegations and the evidence.* (London: Social Affairs Unit, 1989), pp 38-52.

Heather, N., 'The Public Health and Brief Interventions for Excessive Alcohol Consumption: The British Experience', *Addictive Behaviours,* 21 (1996), pp 857-868.

Hesketh, T., *The Second Partitioning of Ireland: The Abortion Referendum of 1983.* (Dublin: Brandsma Books, 1990).

Higgins, J., *The Business of Medicine: Private Health Care in Britain.* (London: Macmillan Education, 1988).

Hodgson, R., 'The treatment of alcohol problems', *Addiction,* 89 (1994), pp 1529-1534.

Hupkens, C., Knibbe, R. and Drop, M., 'Alcohol Consumption in the European Community: uniformity and diversity in drinking patterns', *Addiction,* 88 (1993), pp 1391-1404.

Illich I., *Limits to Medicine: Medical Nemesis – the Expropriation of Health.* (London: Marion Boyars, 1977).

Irish Council of Churches/Roman Catholic Joint Group on the Role of the Churches in Irish Society, *Report of the Working Party on the Abuse of Drugs.* (Dublin, 1972).

Jellinek, E., 'Phases of Alcohol Addiction', *Quarterly Journal of Studies on Alcohol,* 13 (1952), pp 673-684.

Jellinek, E., *The Disease Concept of Alcoholism.* (New Haven: Hill House Press, 1961).

Johnson, B., *The alcoholism movement in America: A study in cultural innovation.* (Unpublished doctoral dissertation, University of Illinois, Urbana-Champaign, 1973).

Jones, M., *The Therapeutic Community: A New Treatment Method in Psychiatry.* (New York: Basic Books, 1953).

Judson, H., *Heroin Addiction in Britain: What Americans Can Learn from the British Experience.* (New York: Harcourt Brace Jovanovich, 1974).

Kelleher, C., *The Future for Health Promotion.* (Galway: Centre for Health Promotion Studies, University College Galway, 1992).

Kelleher, C., 'Promoting Health' in Robins, J. (ed.), *Reflections on Health: Commemoration of Fifty Years of Health 1947-1997.* (Dublin: Department of Health, 1997), pp 29-40.

Kelly, M., 'Misuse of a Morphine Alternative (Diconal), *Journal of the Irish Medical Association,* 65 (1972), pp 414-415.

Kendell, R., 'Drinking Sensibly', *British Journal of Addiction,* 82 (1987), pp 1279-1288.

Kennedy, J., *The Unmasking of Medicine.* (London: Allen and Unwin, 1981).

Kerrigan, C., *Father Mathew and the Irish Temperance Movement 1838-1849.* (Cork University Press, 1992).

Kickert, W., Klijn, E. and Koppenjan, J., *Managing Complex Networks: Strategies for the Public Service.* (London: Sage, 1997).

King, E., 'HIV Prevention and the New Virology' in Oppenheimer, J. and Reckitt, H. (eds), *Acting on AIDS: Sex, Drugs and Politics.* (London: Serpents Towl, 1997), pp 11-33.

Kurtz, E., *Not God: A History of Alcoholics Anonymous* (expanded ed.). (Center City, Minnesota: Hazelden, 1991).

Lalonde, M., *A New Perspective on the Health of Canadians.* (Ottawa: Information Canada, 1974).

Lee, J., 'Centralisation and Community' in Lee, J. (ed.), *Ireland: Towards a Sense of Place.* (Cork University Press, 1985), pp 84-101.

Lee, J., *Ireland 1912-1985: Politics and Society.* (Cambridge University Press, 1989).

Levine, H.G., 'Temperance Cultures: concerns about alcohol problems in Nordic and English-speaking countries' in Lader, M., Edwards, G. and Drummond, D.C. (eds), *The Nature of Alcohol and Drug Related Problems.* (Oxford University Press, 1992), pp 15-36.

Levine, H.G., and Reinarman, C., 'From Prohibition to Regulation: Lessons from Alcohol Policy for Drug Policy' in Bayer, R. and Oppenheimer, G. (eds), *Confronting Drug Policy: Illicit Drugs in a Free Society.* (New York: Cambridge University Press, 1993), pp 162-178.

Lewis, A., 'Health as a Social Concept', *British Journal of Sociology,* 4 (1953), pp 107-115.

Lindesmith, A., *Opiate Addiction.* (Bloomington Indiana: Principia Press, 1947).

Macken, U., *Drug Abuse in Ireland.* (Cork: Mercier Press, 1975).

Makela, K., et al, *Alcoholics Anonymous as a Mutual-Help Movement: A Study in Eight Societies.* (University of Wisconsin Press, 1996).

Makela, K., et al, *Alcohol, Society and the State (Vol. 1): A Comparative Study of Alcohol Control.* (Toronto: Addiction Research Foundation, 1981).

Malcolm, E., *Ireland Sober, Ireland Free: Drink and Temperance in Nineteenth-Century Ireland.* (Dublin: Gill and Macmillan, 1986).

Malcolm, E., *Swift's Hospital: A History of St. Patrick's Hospital Dublin 1746-1989.* (Dublin: Gill and Macmillan, 1989).

Malone, P., 'Community Action in the North Inner City' in O'Donohue, N. and Richardson, S., *Pure Murder: A Book about Drug Use.* (Dublin: Women's Community Press, 1984), pp 75-81.

Manly, D., Browne, L., Cox, G. and Lowry, P., *The Facilitators.* (Dublin: Brandsma Books, 1986).

Mann, J., '... for a global challenge', *World Health* (March 1988), pp 3-5.

Martin, W., 'Concerned Parents Against Drugs Action Group' in O'Donohue, N. and Richardson, S. (eds), *Pure Murder: A Book about Drug Use.* (Dublin: Women's Community Press, 1984), pp 71-75.

MacGregor, S., 'Medicine, Custom or Moral Fibre: Policy Responses to Drug Misuse' in N. South (ed.), *Drugs: Cultures, Controls and Everyday Life.* (London: Sage, 1999), pp 67-85.

McCann, M.E., *Ten Years On: A history of the Ballymun Youth Action Project, a community response to drug and alcohol abuse.* (Ballymun Youth Action Project, 1991).

McCarrroll, J., *Is the School Around the Corner Just the Same?* (Dublin: Brandsma Books, 1987).

McCoy, D., *Issues for Irish Alcohol Policy: A Historical Perspective with Some Lessons for the Future.* (Paper read before the Statistical and Social Inquiry Society of Ireland, 24 October, 1991).

McKinsey and Co., *Towards Better Health Care Management in the Health Boards (Volumes 1 and 2).* (Dublin: Department of Health, 1970/71).

McLernon, C., Bateson, R. and Hynes, M., *Press Coverage of the 1994 Legislative Change in the Drink-Driving Laws in Ireland.* (Dublin Healthy Cities Project, 1995).

McNamara, K., *Curriculum and Values in Education.* (Dublin: Veritas, 1987).

Middleton Fillmore, K., 'Competing Paradigms in Biomedical and Social Science Alcohol Research: The 1940s Through the 1980s' in Roman, P. (ed.), *Alcohol: The Development of Sociological Perspectives on Use and Abuse.* (New Brunswick, New Jersey: Rutgers Center of Alcohol Studies, 1991), pp 59-85.

Milio, N., 'Making healthy public policy; developing the science by learning the art: an ecological framework for policy studies', *Health Promotion,* 2 (1988), pp 263-274.

Miller, W. and Hester, R., 'The effectiveness of alcoholism treatment: what research reveals' in Miller, W. and Heather, N. (eds), *Treating Addictive Behaviors: Processes of Change.* (New York: Plenum Press, 1986), pp 121-174.

Miller, W. and Kurtz, E., 'Models of Alcoholism Used in Treatment; Contrasting AA and other Perspectives With Which It Is Often Confused', *Journal of Studies on Alcohol,* 55 (1994), pp 159-166.

Miller, W. et al, 'What Works? A Methodological Analysis of the Alcohol Treatment Outcome Literature' in Hester, R. and Milller, W. (eds), *Handbook of Alcoholism Treatment Approaches: Effective Alternatives (2nd ed.).* (Boston: Allyn and Bacon, 1995), pp 12-44.

Moos, R., Finney, J. and Cronkite, R., *Alcoholism Treatment: Context, Process and Outcome.* (New York: Oxford University Press, 1990).

Morgan, M. and Grube, J., *Drinking Among Post-Primary School Pupils.* (Dublin: Economic and Social Research Institute, 1994).

Moser, J., 'What does a national alcohol policy look like?' in Glass, I. (ed.), *The International Handbook of Addiction Behaviour.* (London: Tavistock/Routledge, 1991), pp 313-319.

Nace, E., 'Alcoholics Anonymous' in Lowinson, J. et al (eds), *Substance Abuse: A Comprehensive Textbook (2nd ed.).* (Baltimore: Williams and Wilkins, 1992), pp 486-495.

Nadelmann, E., 'Global Prohibition Regimes: the evolution of norms in international society', *International Organisation,* 44 (1990), pp 479-526.

Nadelmann, E., 'US Drug Policy: A Bad Export', *Foreign Policy,* 70 (1988), pp 93-101.

Naidoo, J., 'Limits to Individualism' in Rodmell, S. and Watt, A. (eds), *The Politics of Health Education: Raising the Issues.* (London: Routledge and Kegan Paul, 1986), pp 17-37.

National Alcohol Policy – Ireland. (Dublin: Stationery Office, 1996).

National Economic and Social Council, *Health Services: The Implications of Demographic Changes. (NESC Paper No. 73).* (Dublin: NESC, 1983).

Newby, H., 'Community and Urban Life' in Worsley, P. (ed.), *The New Introducing Sociology.* (London: Penguin Books, 1987), pp 238-272.

Newman, J., *Puppets of Utopia: Can Irish democracy be taken for granted?* (Dublin: Four Courts Press, 1987).

Nutbeam, D., Blakey, V. and Pates, R., 'The Prevention of HIV Infection from Injecting Drug Use – A Review of Health Promotion Approaches', *Social Science and Medicine,* 33 (1991), pp 977-983.

Ó Cinnéide, S., 'Democracy and the Constitution', *Administration*, 46 (Winter 1998/99), pp 41-58.

O'Connell, C., 'Tenant Involvement in Local Authority Estate Management: A New Panacea for Policy Failure?', *Administration*, 46, (1998), pp 25-46.

O'Doherty, E.F. and McGrath, S. (eds), *The Priest and Mental Health.* (Dublin: Clonmore and Reynolds, 1962).

O'Donnell, R., 'Irish Policy in a Global Context: From State Autonomy to Social Partnership' in Walsh, J. and Leavy, B., *Strategy and General Management: An Irish Reader.* (Dublin: Oaktreee Press, 1995), pp 299-321.

O'Donohue, N. and Richardson, S., *Pure Murder: A Book about Drug Use.* (Dublin: Women's Community Press, 1984).

O'Hagan, M. and McGovern, T., 'The Alcoholism/Drug Dependency Counsellor, Health Care Professional in the US and Ireland' in *Proceedings of Health for All – Meeting the Challenge.* (Twelfth World Conference on Health Education). (Dublin: Health Education Bureau, 1987), pp 987-988.

O'Halpin, E., 'Policy Making' in Coakley, J. and Gallagher, M. (eds), *Politics in the Republic of Ireland.* (Galway: PSAI Press, 1992), pp 167-181.

O'Hanlon, R., 'Launch Address' in Kelleher, C. (ed.), *The Future for Health Promotion.* (Galway: Centre for Health Promotion Studies, 1992), pp 3-8.

O'Hare, A. and Walsh, D., *Activities of Irish Psychiatric Hospitals and Units 1979.* (Dublin: Medico-Social Research Board, 1981).

O'Hare, P. et al, *The Reduction of Drug Related Harm.* (London: Routledge, 1992).

O'Kelly, F. et al, 'The Rise and Fall of Heroin Use in an Inner City Area of Dublin', *Irish Journal of Medical Science,* 157 (1988), pp 35-38.

O'Mahony, P. and Gilmore, T., *Drug Abusers in the Dublin Committal Prisons: A Survey.* (Dublin: Stationery Office, 1982).

O'Mahony, P. and Smith, E., 'Some Personality Characteristics of Imprisoned Heroin Addicts', *Drug and Alcohol Dependence,* 13 (1984), pp 255-265.

Orford, J. and Edwards, G., *Alcoholism: A Comparison of Treatment and Advice, with the Influence of Marriage.* (Oxford University Press, 1977).

O'Riordan, S., 'Round the Reviews', *The Furrow* (January 1952), pp 31-40.

O'Riordan, S., 'Round the Reviews', *The Furrow* (May 1952), pp 203-210.

O'Riordan, S., 'Alcoholism' in O'Doherty, E.F. and McGrath, S. (eds), *The Priest and Mental Health.* (Dublin: Clonmore and Reynolds, 1962), pp 150-154.

Ottawa Charter for Health Promotion. (Geneva: World Health Organisation, 1986).

Page, P., 'E.M. Jellinek and the evolution of alcohol studies: a critical essay', *Addiction,* 92 (1997), pp 1619-1637.

Parker, H., Aldridge, J. and Measham, F., *Illegal Leisure: The normalization of adolescent recreational drug use.* (London: Routledge, 1998).

Parsons, T., *The Social System.* (London: Routledge and Kegan Paul, 1951).

Peele, S., 'Can Alcoholism and Other Drug Addiction Problems be Treated Away or is the Current Treatment Binge Doing More Harm Than Good?' *Journal of Psycohactive Drugs,* 20 (1988), pp 375-382.

Peele, S., *Diseasing of America: Addiction Treatment out of Control.* (Lexington, Mass.: Lexington Books, 1989).

Perceval, R., *Alcoholism and Drug Abuse.* (Dublin: Veritas, 1970).

Petersen, A. and Lupton, D., *The New Public Health: Health and Self in the Age of Risk.* (London: Sage, 1996).

Philpott, G., *Deep End.* (Dublin: Poolbeg Press, 1995).

Picardie, J. and Wade, J., *Heroin: Chasing the Dragon.* (Penguin Books, 1985).

Pinker, R., 'An alternative view' in *Social Workers: Their Role and Task.* (London: Bedford Square Press, 1982), pp 236-262.

Power, R., 'Drugs and the Media: prevention campaigns and television', in MacGregor, S. (ed.), *Drugs and British Society: Responses to a Social Problem in the 1980s.* (London: Routledge, 1989), pp 129-142.

Promoting Health Through Public Policy. (Dublin: Health Education Bureau, 1987).

Public Services Organisation Review Group. (Dublin: Stationery Office, 1969).

Report of the Commission of Inquiry on Mental Illness. (Dublin: Stationery Office, 1966).

Report of the Commission on Health Funding. (Dublin: Stationery Office, 1989).

Report of the Committee of Inquiry into the Drugs Problem in the Member States of the Community. (Strasbourg: European Parliament, 1985).

Report of the Committee on Drug Education. (Dublin: Stationery Office, 1974).

Report of the Expert Group on the establishment of a Protocol for the Prescribing of Methadone. (Dublin: Department of Health, 1993).

Report of the Inspector of Mental Hospitals for the Year ending 31 December 1992. (Dublin: Stationery Office, 1995).

Report of the Intoxicating Liquor Commission. (Dublin: Stationery Office, 1925).

Report of the Working Party on Drug Abuse. (Dublin: Stationery Office, 1971).

Reynolds, J., *Grangegorman: Psychiatric Care in Dublin since 1815.* (Dublin: Institute of Public Administration, 1992).

Rhodes, T., *Outreach work with drug users: principles and practice.* (Strasbourg: Council of Europe, 1996).

Robins, J., *Fools and Mad.* (Dublin: Institute of Public Administration, 1986).

Robinson, D., 'The Alcohologist's Addiction', *Quarterly Journal of Studies on Alcohol,* 33 (1972), pp 908-916.

Room, R., *Governing Images of Alcohol and Drug Problems.* (Unpublished PhD Dissertation, University of California, Berkeley, 1978).

Ross, H., *Confronting Drunk Driving: Social Policy for Saving Lives.* (Yale University Press, 1992).

Royal College of Psychiatrists, *Alcohol: Our Favourite Drug.* (London: Tavistock, 1986).

Schur, E., *Narcotic addiction in Britain and America: the impact of public policy.* (London: Associated Book Publishers, 1966).

Secker, A., 'The policy-research interface: an insider's view', *Addiction,* 88 (1993), pp 1195-1205.

Seeley, J., 'Alcoholism as a Disease: Implications for Social Policy' in Pittman, D. and Snyder, C. (eds), *Society, Culture and Drinking Problems.* (New York: John Wiley, 1962), pp 592-599.

Shadwell, A., *Drink in 1914-1922: A Lesson in Control.* (New York: Longmans Green and Co., 1923).

Shaping a Healthier Future: A Strategy for Effective Healthcare in the 1990s. (Dublin: Stationery Office, 1994).

Shaw, S., 'A Critique of the Concept of the Alcohol Dependence Syndrome', *British Journal of Addiction,* 74 (1979), pp 339-348.

Shaw, S., Cartwright, A., Spratley, T. and Harwin, J., *Responding to Drinking Problems.* (London: Croom Helm, 1978).

Shilts, R., *And the Band Played On: People, Politics and the AIDS Epidemic.* (Penguin, 1988).

Single, E. et al, *Alcohol, Society and the State (vol. 2): The Social History of Control Policy in Seven Countries.* (Toronto: Addiction Research Foundation, 1981).

Single, E., 'Defining harm reduction', *Drug and Alcohol Review,* 14 (1995), pp 287-290.

Skranabek, P., 'Preventive Medicine and Morality', *The Lancet (i)* 1986, pp 144-145.

Skrabanek, P., 'Nonsensus Consensus', *The Lancet,* 335 (1990), pp 1446-1447.

Smyth, R., Keenan, E., Dorman, A. and O'Connor, J., 'Hepatitis C Infection among Injecting Drug Users attending the National Drug Treatment Centre', *Irish Journal of Medical Science,* 164 (1995), pp 267-268.

Stevenson, R. and Carney, A., 'Social and Psychological Characteristics of Drug Addicts Interviewed in Dublin', *Irish Medical Journal,* 4 (1971), pp 372-375.

Stimson, G., Donoghue, M., Hart, R. and Dolan, K., 'Distributing Sterile Needles and Syringes to People who Inject Drugs: The Syringe-Exchange Experiment', in Strang, J. and Stimson, G. (eds), *AIDS and Drug Misuse: The Challenge for Policy and Practice in the 1990s.* (London: Routledge, 1990), pp 222-231.

Stimson, G. and Lart, R., 'The relationship between the State and local practice in the development of national policy on drugs between 1920 and 1990', in Strang, J. and Gossop, M. (eds), *Heroin Addiction and Drug Policy: The British System.* (Oxford University Press, 1994), pp 331-341.

Strang, J., 'A model service: turning the generalist on to drugs', in MacGregor, S. (ed.), *Drugs and British Society: Responses to a social problem in the 1980s.* (London: Routledge, 1989), pp 143-169.

Strang, J., 'The British System: past, present and future', *International Review of Psychiatry,* 1 (1990), pp 109-120.

Strang, J. and Clement, S., 'The introduction of Community Drug Teams Across the UK' in Strang, J. and Gossop, M. (eds), *Heroin Addiction and Drug Policy: The British System.* (Oxford University Press, 1994), pp 207-221.

Szasz, T., *Ceremonial Chemistry: The Ritual Persecution of Drugs, Drug Addicts and Pushers.* (London: Routledge and Kegan Paul, 1975).

The Psychiatric Services: Planning for the Future. (Dublin: Stationery Office, 1984).

The Task Force to Review Services for Drug Misusers: Report of an Independent Survey of Drug Treatment Services in England. (Wetherby: Department of Health, 1996).

Trautman, F. and Barendregt, C., *The European Peer Support Project: Development and Encouragement of Peer Support Initiatives for AIDS Prevention in IDU Communities.* (Utrecht: National Institute for Alcohol and Drugs, 1996).

Trebach, A., *The Heroin Solution.* (Yale University Press, 1982).

Vaillant, G., *The Natural History of Alcoholism.* (Harvard University Press, 1983).

Vaillant, G., *The Natural History of Alcoholism Revisited.* (Harvard University Press, 1995).

Walsh, B., *Drinking in Ireland.* (Dublin: Economic and Social Research Institute, 1980).

Walsh, D., 'Alcohol and Alcohol Problems Research 15 – Ireland', *British Journal of Addiction,* 82 (1987), pp 747-751

Walsh, D., 'Alcohol and Ireland', *British Journal of Addiction,* 82 (1987), pp 119-122.

Walsh, D., 'Alcoholism and the Irish', *The Journal of Alcoholism,* 7 (1972).

Walsh, D. and Walsh, B., 'Drowning the Shamrock: Alcohol and Drink in Ireland' in Single, E. et al, *Alcohol, Society and the State (vol. 1): A Comparative History of Control Policy in Seven Countries.* (Toronto: Addiction Research Foundation, 1981).

Wegscheider, S., *Another Chance: Hope and Health for the Alcoholic Family.* (Palo Alto: Science and Behaviour Books, 1981).

Weisner, C. and Room, R., 'Financing and Ideology in Alcohol Treatment', *Social Problems,* 32 (1984), pp 167-184.

Whyte, J., *Church and State in Modern Ireland, 1923-1979* (2nd ed.). (Dublin: Gill and Macmillan, 1980).

Wiener, R., *Drugs and Schoolchildren.* (London: Longman, 1970).

Wiley, M., 'Health Expenditure Trends in Ireland: Past, Present and Future', in Leahy, A. and Wiley, M. (eds), *The Irish Health System in the 21st Century.* (Dublin: Oak Tree Press 1998), pp 69-82.

Williams, G. and Poppay, J., 'Lay knowledge and the privilege of experience' in Gabe, J., Kelleher, D. and Williams, G. (eds), *Challenging Medicine.* (London: Routledge, 1994), pp 118-134.

Wilson-Schaef, A., *Co-Dependence: Misunderstood – Mistreated.* (San Francisco: Harper, 1986).

Woititz, J., *Adult Children of Alcoholics.* (Florida: Health Communications Inc., 1990).

World Health Organisation, *Ottawa Charter for Health Promotion.* (Geneva: WHO, 1986).

World Health Organisation, *Primary Health Care (Report of the International Conference on Primary Health Care, Alma Ata, 6-12 September 1978).* (Geneva: WHO, 1978).

World Health Organisation, *WHO Expert Committee on Mental Health Alcoholism Sub-committee, 2nd report (WHO Technical Report Series No. 48).* (Geneva: WHO, 1952).

World Health Organisation, *WHO Expert Committee on Problems Related to Alcohol and Consumption. (WHO Technical Report Series No. 650).* (Geneva: WHO, 1980).

Yablonsky, L., *The Tunnel Back: Synanon.* (New York: Macmillan, 1965).

Young, J., *The Drugtakers: The Social Meaning of Drug Use.* (London: Paladin, 1971).

Zola, I., 'Medicine as an Institution of Social Control', *Sociological Review,* 20 (1973), pp 487-504.

Index

versus disease concept of alcoholism
44-74

R
Rabbitte, Pat 201
Rabbitte Report 201-5, 223, 225
Rainbow Coalition 95
Reagan, Nancy 166
Reagan, Ronald 166
rehabilitation 1
*Report of the Commission of Inquiry on
Mental Illness* 37, 38, 109
*Report of the Inspector of Mental
Hospitals for 1958* 46
*Report of the Inspector of Mental
Hospitals for 1992* 100
*Report of the Working Party on Drug
Abuse* 158, 189
Revenue Commissioners 9, 45
Road Traffic Act 1994 92, 94, 95, 97,
103, 213
Rockefeller Institute, New York 108
Roman Catholic Church
and Alcoholics Anonymous 25-8
and drugs 179
influence on social policy 12, 14
and licensing laws 30-1, 33, 39-40
and Minnesota Model 55-6
and Pioneer Total Abstinence
Association 19
Room, Robin 21, 47
Ross, Shane 67
Rossmore, Lord Paddy 126
RTÉ 199
Rutland Centre 56-8
Ryan, Brendan 144
Ryan, Dr John 120

S
Seán McDermott Street area 151,
154-7
Seanad 33
Secker, A. 68-9, 70
Seeley, J. 46
Select Dáil Committee on Legislation
and Security 87
self-help 12-13

Shaping a Healthier Future 7-8, 84, 95,
98-9
Shatter, Alan 67
Sheils, Gertie 93, 95-6
Short, Fr Raphael 56-7, 58, 59
Single Convention on Narcotic Drugs
1961 129
Sinn Féin 161
Skrabanek, P. 14, 15
Smith, Michael 92, 94
Smith, Patricia 152
social partnership 12, 203
socio-economic disadvantage, and drug
addiction 116-17, 125-6, 128,
131, 134, 140, 143-4, 146, 150-2,
158-9, 202
Southern Health Board 216
Special Governmental Task Force on
Drug Abuse 140-2, 145-6, 156,
180, 202-3
Special Hospital (Mental Health)
Programme 147-8
St Brendan's Hospital, St Dymphna's in-
patient addiction unit 120-1, 123
St Brigid's Hospital, Ballinasloe 101
St Dymphna's Hospital 53, 57
St John of God's Hospital 101
St Lawrence's Hospital 57
St Mary's Hospital, Minneapolis 56
St Patrick's College, Maynooth 27
St Patrick's Hospital 25, 34, 36, 54, 60
St Teresa's Gardens 151-7, 165
Stanhope Social Service Centre 56, 61
Stanhope Street Alcoholism Centre 61
*Statistical and Social Inquiry Society of
Ireland* 19
Stevenson, Dr R.D. 53, 57, 65, 120, 123
Strategic Management Initiative 11, 20,
25, 203
*Strategy for Health for All by the Year
2000* 4, 6
structure of book 16-17
Sunday Business Post 199
Sunday Tribune 94
Sweden 216
Synanon 126
Szasz, T. 16